RURAL ORTHOPEDIC EMERGENCY POCKET GUIDE

DR. MOHAMED ELGENDY, LMCC, CCFP, CANADA

DISCLAIMER

This pocket guide was developed with the assistance of advanced AI tools to streamline content generation. Every chapter has been thoroughly reviewed, edited, and authenticated by Dr. Mohamed Elgendy, LMCC, CCFP (Canada), ensuring accuracy, credibility, and clinical authenticity. The result is a modern, innovative reference that blends the efficiency of AI with the rigor of professional medical expertise

This booklet summarizes orthopedic emergency care principles based on publicly available clinical guidelines and practice statements. It does not reproduce proprietary tables, figures, algorithms, or distinctive wording from subscription-only sources. Content is for education and exam preparation; it is not a substitute for clinical judgment, institutional policies, or local protocols.

Clinical responsibility remains with the treating clinician. Always consult current local guidelines, official product monographs, and institutional pathways. Verify drug doses and contraindications with authoritative sources prior to use.

ABOUT THE AUTHOR

Dr. Mohamed Elgendy is a licensed Canadian physician with the Licentiate of the Medical Council of Canada (LMCC) and Certification in Family Medicine (CCFP) from the College of Family Physicians of Canada. He has several years of hands-on experience as both a rural emergency physician and a family doctor, currently practicing in Saskatchewan, Canada. With a deep commitment to improving healthcare delivery in underserved communities, Dr. Elgendy focuses on practical, evidence-based medicine tailored to the realities of rural practice. His work bridges the gap between academic medicine and frontline care, offering accessible resources to help clinicians make confident, life-saving decisions in resource-limited settings

DEDICATION

This book is dedicated to the patients in rural and remote communities, whose strength and perseverance inspire every effort; to the healthcare providers who manage orthopedic emergencies with skill, compassion, and resourcefulness in the face of limited resources; and to my family, whose constant support makes this work possible.

— Dr. Mohamed Elgendy

TABLE OF CONTENTS

PROTOCOLS, DECISION-MAKING & COMMUNICATION

CHAPTER 1
Trauma Protocol (ABCDE) – Orthopedic Considerations in Rural Emergency Care

Introduction

The standard trauma approach using the ABCDE framework (Airway, Breathing, Circulation, Disability, Exposure) applies equally in rural emergency settings. However, orthopedic injuries may influence or complicate each step. This chapter outlines how to incorporate orthopedic awareness into each phase of the trauma protocol.

A – Airway with Cervical Spine Protection

1. Assess airway patency while maintaining C-spine precautions
2. Assume C-spine injury in any high-velocity trauma, especially with upper extremity fractures or maxillofacial injuries
3. Apply rigid cervical collar and use jaw-thrust maneuver
4. Prepare for intubation in patients with flail chest, severe pain, or altered LOC

B – Breathing

1. Assess chest expansion, auscultate breath sounds
2. Look for rib fractures, flail chest, or pneumothorax
3. Tension pneumothorax may be masked by distracting orthopedic injuries
4. Immobilize upper limb fractures to reduce splinting and improve ventilation
5. Treat pain aggressively to prevent hypoventilation

C – Circulation with Hemorrhage Control

1. Check pulses, control external bleeding from open fractures
2. Apply pressure, hemostatic dressing, or tourniquet if needed
3. Assess for pelvic fractures—apply pelvic binder early in suspected unstable pelvis
4. Monitor for signs of hypovolemia (tachycardia, hypotension)
5. IV access above injury level; fluid resuscitate as needed

D – Disability (Neurologic Status)

1. Assess GCS, pupils, limb strength and sensation
2. Rule out spinal cord injury in patients with long bone fractures and altered sensation
3. Check for compartment syndrome (5 P's) regularly
4. Document distal neurovascular status before and after splinting or reduction

E – Exposure and Environmental Control

1. Fully expose patient to assess for hidden injuries
2. Look for limb deformity, open wounds, or missed fractures
3. Avoid hypothermia: warm fluids, blankets, heat lamps
4. Document orthopedic injuries clearly with side, type, and suspected fracture classification

Orthopedic Pearls in Trauma

1. Prioritize life-threatening injuries before limb salvage
2. Suspect femur fractures and pelvic fractures as sources of major blood loss

3. Early splinting of long bone fractures reduces pain, bleeding, and complications
4. Open fractures = orthopedic emergency – start IV antibiotics within 1 hour
5. Document NV exam before/after any intervention

CHAPTER 2
Open Fractures – Rural Emergency Management and Transfer Protocol

Introduction

Open fractures involve direct communication between a fractured bone and the external environment, increasing the risk of infection, nonunion, and complications. They are orthopedic emergencies requiring early antibiotics, tetanus prophylaxis, and urgent surgical debridement. Rural physicians must act promptly to stabilize and transfer.

Assessment

Key Signs:

1. Visible bone through the wound
2. Wound near fracture with bubbling, air, or fat globules
3. Contaminated wounds (e.g., farm injuries, water exposure)
4. High-energy mechanism or penetrating injury

Assess for:

1. Neurovascular compromise (document motor/sensory/pulses)
2. Size and contamination of the wound
3. Associated injuries (e.g., compartment syndrome, tendon injury)
4. Degree of soft tissue damage

Management

Immediate Management:

1. Control bleeding with direct pressure
2. Cover wound with sterile moist dressing (do NOT probe or irrigate extensively)
3. Immobilize limb with splint
4. IV antibiotics ASAP (ideally within 1 hour):
5. Cefazolin 2 g IV q8h
6. Add Gentamicin 5–7 mg/kg IV for Type III or heavily contaminated wounds
7. Add Penicillin G 4 million units IV q4h if farm injury (Clostridium concern)

Tetanus prophylaxis:

1. If unknown or >10 years, give Td or Tdap
2. Consider tetanus immune globulin (TIG) if not previously immunized

Do not close wound in rural ED — leave open and covered with sterile gauze

When to Refer

Immediate Transfer:

1. All open fractures, regardless of size or contamination
2. Suspected vascular or nerve injury
3. Contaminated wounds (e.g., water, soil, feces)
4. Farm or crush injuries
5. Any open joint injury

Call receiving facility, document timing of:

1. Injury
2. Antibiotic administration
3. Neurovascular exams before and after splinting

Admission Orders

1. Admit to Rural Medicine – Open Fracture Stabilization and Transfer
2. Diagnosis: [e.g., Open midshaft tibial fracture – Gustilo II]
3. Condition: Critical
4. Allergies: [Document here]

Orders:

1. Vitals q1h, monitor NV status q1h
2. NPO
3. IV NS at 100 mL/h

Antibiotics:

1. Cefazolin 2 g IV q8h
2. Gentamicin 5 mg/kg IV once (if needed)
3. Penicillin G 4 MU IV q4h (if farm injury)
4. Tetanus toxoid 0.5 mL IM
5. Tetanus immune globulin 250 units IM (if indicated)
6. Cover wound with sterile moist gauze
7. Immobilize with splint
8. Analgesia: Morphine 2–4 mg IV q4h PRN
9. CBC, Cr, Lytes, INR/PTT, Group & Screen
10. Arrange urgent surgical transfer – contact ortho at receiving hospital

Rural ER Pearls

1. Antibiotics are the most important early intervention — give within 1 hour.
2. Never close the wound or probe it in the ED.
3. Use a moist sterile dressing and immobilize before transfer.
4. Tetanus prophylaxis should not be overlooked — document status clearly.
5. Early ortho involvement improves outcomes — make the call early.

CHAPTER 3
Safe Discharge vs Admission vs Transfer – Decision-Making in Rural Orthopedic Emergencies

Introduction

In rural emergency medicine, deciding whether a patient with an orthopedic injury can be safely discharged, requires admission, or needs transfer to a higher-level facility is a critical skill. This decision must consider patient safety, available resources, injury severity, and access to follow-up care.

Safe for Discharge – Criteria and Cases

Discharge Criteria:

1. Stable vital signs
2. No neurovascular compromise
3. Adequate pain control with oral medications
4. Patient or caregiver able to manage splint care and follow-up
5. Safe environment for recovery
6. Clear follow-up arranged (e.g., ortho clinic, family doctor)

Examples:

1. Minor sprains or stable nondisplaced fractures (e.g., toe, finger, radial head)
2. Closed reduction of shoulder dislocation with good neurovascular status
3. Simple metacarpal fracture treated with gutter splint
4. Minor soft tissue injuries with normal imaging

9

Discharge Instructions:

1. Elevation, icing, and splint care
2. Signs of compartment syndrome or infection
3. Analgesia regimen and stool softener
4. Follow-up appointment within 1 week

Indications for Admission

Admit If:

1. Pain uncontrolled with oral meds
2. Patient unable to manage ADLs or self-care
3. High-risk social situation (e.g., elder abuse, cognitive impairment, no home support)
4. Requires IV antibiotics (e.g., open fracture, cellulitis around injury)
5. Needs scheduled OR but cannot transfer same day

Common Examples:

1. Elderly patient with pubic rami fracture and mobility issues
2. Septic joint pending OR
3. Open fracture stabilized but delayed transfer
4. Limb-threatening ischemia under observation awaiting surgery

Admission Orders:

1. Vital signs q4h, neurovascular checks
2. IV fluids, analgesia (e.g., morphine PRN)
3. Antibiotics if indicated (e.g., cefazolin)
4. NPO if surgical plan pending
5. Ortho consult and daily reassessment

Indications for Urgent Transfer

Transfer Immediately If:

1. Compartment syndrome
2. Open fracture requiring urgent OR
3. Neurovascular compromise
4. Unstable pelvic or femur fracture
5. Septic joint
6. Irreducible dislocation
7. Pediatric Salter-Harris III–V
8. Lack of resources for monitoring or imaging

Before Transfer:

1. Stabilize fracture (splint), IV access, tetanus, analgesia, antibiotics
2. Document NV status pre- and post-intervention
3. Call receiving center and transport agency (e.g., STARS, RAAPID)
4. Provide verbal and written handover

Documentation Essentials

1. Mechanism and timing of injury
2. NV status and pain scores before/after interventions
3. Sedation and reduction attempts
4. Rationale for discharge, admission, or transfer
5. Specific instructions given to patient or caregiver
6. Follow-up details or receiving hospital/physician

Rural ER Pearls

1. Always consider the patient's home situation and transport barriers.
2. Don't discharge if you wouldn't be comfortable treating the same injury at home without help.
3. When in doubt, discuss with on-call orthopedic or use regional consultation lines.
4. Arrange follow-up before discharge when possible.

CHAPTER 4
When to Call Orthopedics Immediately – Red Flags in Rural Emergency Orthopedic Care

Introduction

Prompt recognition of orthopedic emergencies requiring immediate consultation or transfer is essential in the rural ER. Delays in referral can lead to irreversible complications including limb loss, joint destruction, and permanent disability. This chapter outlines high-risk orthopedic scenarios that require urgent orthopedic input.

Situations Requiring Immediate Ortho Consultation or Transfer

1. Open Fractures

- Fractures with communication to the external environment
- High infection risk and need for urgent surgical washout

2. Neurovascular Compromise

- Absent pulses, pallor, paresthesia, paralysis, or pain out of proportion
- Common in dislocations, supracondylar fractures, tibial plateau fractures

3. Compartment Syndrome

- Pain out of proportion, pain on passive stretch, pulselessness, pallor, paresthesia, paralysis
- Requires emergent fasciotomy

4. Irreducible Dislocations

- Inability to perform closed reduction despite adequate sedation
- Indicates soft tissue interposition or fracture entrapment

5. Septic Joint

- Suspected or confirmed joint infection
- Requires emergent aspiration, antibiotics, and operative washout

6. Acute Hip Dislocation

- Often seen in prosthetic hips or trauma
- Time-sensitive to reduce risk of avascular necrosis

7. Pediatric Growth Plate Injuries (Salter-Harris III–V)

- May require precise reduction to prevent growth arrest

8. Spinal Fractures with Neurologic Signs

- Immediate neurosurgical or orthopedic spinal input needed
- Immobilize and transfer urgently

9. Fat Embolism Syndrome

- Seen in long bone fractures (femur, pelvis)
- Respiratory distress, petechiae, altered mental status – requires ICU transfer

10. Floating Knee or Elbow Injuries

- Simultaneous fractures above and below a joint
- Often unstable with vascular concerns

Other High-Risk Situations for Urgent Ortho Advice

1. Displaced intra-articular fractures
2. Unstable pelvic fractures
3. Tendon ruptures with functional loss (e.g., quadriceps, Achilles)
4. Pathologic fractures (e.g., in cancer or cysts)
5. Traumatic amputations or mangled extremity

Rural ER Protocol

1. Stabilize the patient (ABCs, splint, analgesia, tetanus, antibiotics)
2. Take initial imaging before calling (if does not delay care)
3. Clearly communicate findings, stability, neurovascular status
4. Use provincial transfer network (e.g., STARS, ORNGE, RAAPID)
5. Document all communication and rationale for transfer

Documentation Essentials

1. Time of injury and presentation
2. Neurovascular status pre- and post-reduction/splint
3. Sedation and analgesia given
4. Imaging performed and interpretation
5. Name and facility of orthopedic consultant contacted
6. Transfer arrangements and time initiated

CHAPTER 5
Orthopedic Referral Note Essentials – Clear, Effective Communication from the Rural ER

Introduction

When referring orthopedic patients from a rural emergency department, a concise and complete referral note ensures continuity of care, reduces medical errors, and facilitates appropriate triage by the receiving orthopedic team. This chapter outlines the essential components of an orthopedic referral note and provides tips for efficient documentation.

Core Components of an Ortho Referral Note

1. Patient Demographics

- Full name, date of birth, health card number
- Contact information and home address

2. Mechanism of Injury

- Describe clearly (e.g., fall from ladder, MVC, sports injury)
- Include time and location of injury

3. Clinical Findings

- Injury site and side (e.g., right distal radius)
- Neurovascular exam before and after intervention
- Swelling, deformity, open wounds

4. Imaging and Interpretation

- X-ray findings (fracture type, displacement, joint involvement)
- CT/MRI (if done) – include report or key findings

- Note if imaging not available or pending

5. Emergency Management Done

- Reduction (if attempted), sedation used
- Splint or immobilization type
- Pain control measures (meds, blocks)
- Tetanus, antibiotics given if indicated

6. Disposition and Reason for Referral

- Clearly state whether patient is stable or unstable
- Why ortho referral is required (e.g., open fracture, needs OR)
- Whether transfer is urgent, semi-urgent, or routine

7. Follow-Up/Transfer Plan

- Any appointments arranged
- Method and time of transfer (if applicable)
- Contact with receiving team or hospital

8. Physician Info and Contact

- Referring doctor's name and facility
- Contact number for clarification or updates

Template for a Rural Ortho Referral Note

Patient Name: John Doe

DOB: Jan 1, 1965

HIN:1234-567-890

Mechanism: Fall off 6-ft ladder while cleaning gutters at 11:00 AM

Injury: Left midshaft tibial fracture, closed

NV Exam: Intact before and after splinting

X-ray: Transverse midshaft tibial fracture, no fibular involvement

Management: Immobilized in long leg posterior splint; given morphine + Tylenol #3

Tetanus: Up to date

Disposition: Requires ORIF; rural OR unavailable

Referral To: Dr. Smith, Ortho at Regina General Hospital

Transfer via: EMS arranged for 6 PM

Referring MD: Dr. Elgendy, Pinewood ER, Tel: (306) 123-4567

Common Pitfalls to Avoid

1. Omitting NV status documentation
2. Incomplete imaging interpretation
3. Not stating urgency of referral
4. No contact number for clarification
5. Poor handwriting or illegible fax/email

ASSESSMENT & PROCEDURAL SKILLS

CHAPTER 6
Analgesia and Sedation in Orthopedic Injuries – Rural Emergency Approach

Introduction

Pain control in orthopedic injuries is crucial for patient comfort, reduction success, and stabilization prior to transfer. In rural emergency settings, physicians must be equipped to provide safe and effective analgesia and procedural sedation, tailored to the available resources and the clinical context.

Initial Pain Management

Non-Pharmacological Measures:

1. Immobilization (splints, slings)
2. Elevation of the limb
3. Ice packs (20 minutes every 2–3 hours)

First-Line Pharmacologic Options:

1. Acetaminophen 650–1000 mg PO q6h PRN
2. Ibuprofen 400–600 mg PO q6–8h PRN (unless contraindicated)
3. Naproxen 250–500 mg PO BID
4. Topical NSAIDs for minor sprains (e.g., diclofenac gel)

Moderate to Severe Pain:

1. Morphine 2.5–5 mg IV q5–10 min PRN (titrate to pain)
2. Hydromorphone 0.5–1 mg IV q10 min PRN
3. Fentanyl 50–100 mcg IV q5 min PRN (shorter duration, rapid onset)

4. Consider oral opioids (e.g., hydromorphone 1–2 mg PO q4–6h) if IV access not available

Procedural Sedation in Orthopedic Reductions

Indications:

1. Closed fracture or dislocation reductions
2. Painful manipulations (e.g., joint relocation)
3. Splinting of unstable fractures

Agents:

1. Ketamine

- Dose: 1–1.5 mg/kg IV (or 3–5 mg/kg IM)
- Onset: 30 seconds; Duration: 10–20 min
- Preserves airway reflexes
- Emergence reactions possible (minimize with midazolam)

2. Midazolam + Fentanyl

- Midazolam 0.05–0.1 mg/kg IV (max 2.5–5 mg)
- Fentanyl 1 mcg/kg IV (max 100 mcg)
- Monitor for respiratory depression

3. Propofol

- 0.5–1 mg/kg IV slow push
- Rapid onset, short duration
- Requires airway and respiratory monitoring
- Not ideal in unstable or hypotensive patients

Monitoring:

1. Cardiac monitor, pulse oximetry, oxygen at bedside
2. Suction and airway equipment ready

3. Atropine, naloxone, and flumazenil available

Regional and Local Techniques

Hematoma Block (e.g., distal radius)

1. 5–10 mL lidocaine 1% without epinephrine
2. Inject directly into fracture hematoma
3. Wait 5–10 minutes before reduction

Bier Block (Intravenous regional anesthesia – distal upper limb)

1. Requires tourniquet and IV access in injured limb
2. 40 mL of 0.5% lidocaine (max 3 mg/kg)
3. Monitor for LAST (local anesthetic systemic toxicity)

Nerve Blocks

1. Digital block (finger injuries): lidocaine 1% 2–3 mL per side
2. Femoral nerve block: 15–20 mL of bupivacaine 0.25% under guidance
3. Ensure no contraindications to local anesthetics (e.g., allergy, severe liver dysfunction)

Discharge and Follow-Up Pain Control

1. Provide clear instructions for home analgesia (acetaminophen + NSAIDs)
2. Warn about opioid side effects (constipation, drowsiness)
3. Provide stool softeners with opioids (e.g., docusate sodium 100 mg BID)
4. Counsel on avoiding driving or machinery under sedation/opiates
5. Arrange timely follow-up for reassessment or specialist review

Rural ER Pearls

1. Always assess and document pain scale (0–10) before and after intervention.
2. Combine immobilization + medications for optimal pain control.
3. Ketamine is excellent for short orthopedic procedures in resource-limited settings.
4. Have a "crash cart" ready during any procedural sedation.
5. Consider nerve blocks to reduce opioid use and facilitate transport

CHAPTER 7
Fracture Reduction Techniques – A Practical Guide for Rural Emergency Physicians

Introduction

Fracture reduction is often necessary in rural emergency departments to relieve pain, restore anatomy, reduce neurovascular compromise, and facilitate safe transfer. While definitive fixation is performed at tertiary centers, rural physicians must be familiar with basic closed reduction techniques and safe immobilization methods.

General Principles of Reduction

1. Always assess neurovascular status before and after reduction.
2. Provide adequate analgesia and sedation (e.g., ketamine, fentanyl/midazolam, local nerve blocks).
3. Use appropriate assistants and patient positioning.
4. Gentle, sustained traction is the cornerstone of reduction.
5. Post-reduction immobilization and imaging are essential.

Pain Management Options:

1. Procedural sedation (e.g., ketamine 1 mg/kg IV)
2. Hematoma block (e.g., 10 mL lidocaine 1% without epi)
3. Regional blocks (e.g., Bier block for distal upper limb)

Reduction Techniques by Fracture Type

1. Colles' Fracture (Distal Radius)

- Apply traction with wrist in slight extension.
- Push distal fragment dorsally and proximally.

24

- Immobilize in sugar tong or volar splint with wrist neutral.

2. Ankle Fracture-Dislocation

- Longitudinal traction at heel with knee flexed
- Correct medial/lateral shift
- Immobilize in posterior slab + stirrup

3. Shoulder Dislocation

- Traction-countertraction (sheet method)
- External rotation method
- Stimson (gravity) method: patient prone with weight on arm

4. Elbow Dislocation

- Flex elbow to 90°, apply longitudinal traction with downward pressure on olecranon
- Immobilize at 90° elbow flexion

5. Hip Dislocation (posterior)

- Allis technique (requires sedation + 2 assistants)
- Longitudinal traction in supine position with hip/knee at 90°

6. Finger Dislocation

- Axial traction followed by hyperextension and reduction
- Buddy tape or dorsal splint

7. Pediatric Forearm Fractures

- Traction with countertraction
- Correct angulation with gentle pressure
- Use sugar tong splint

Post-Reduction Care

1. Reassess pulses, cap refill, sensation, and motor function
2. Apply appropriate splint (see Splinting chapter)
3. Elevate limb and provide ice
4. Post-reduction X-rays to confirm alignment
5. Provide written and verbal discharge instructions if not transferring
6. Document reduction method, sedation used, and neurovascular findings before/after

When to Refer

Urgent Transfer:

1. Inability to reduce fracture/dislocation
2. Persistent neurovascular compromise after reduction
3. Open fractures
4. Complex intra-articular fractures
5. Stabilize first, then call receiving facility. Send imaging, reduction note, and sedation records.

Rural ER Pearls

1. Closed reduction can greatly reduce pain and swelling prior to transport.
2. Never force a reduction — use traction and patience.
3. Ensure adequate sedation and monitoring.
4. Practice techniques regularly with simulation.
5. Document thoroughly to protect both patient and physician.

CHAPTER 8
Immobilization and Splinting Techniques

Introduction

Immobilization and splinting are essential skills in rural emergency medicine to stabilize orthopedic injuries, provide pain relief, and prevent further damage. In resource-limited settings, the ability to apply effective and safe splints can greatly influence patient outcomes before transfer or follow-up.

Assessment

Indications:

1. Suspected fractures
2. Joint dislocations (pre/post-reduction)
3. Ligament injuries and tendon ruptures
4. Immobilization prior to transfer
5. Pain control and soft tissue rest

Assessment Prior to Splinting:

1. History of injury and mechanism
2. Neurovascular status (before and after)
3. Deformity, swelling, open wounds
4. Radiographic confirmation when possible

Materials Needed:

1. Plaster or fiberglass splinting material
2. Padding (webril, stockinette)
3. Elastic bandage or tape
4. Scissors, gloves, water for plaster

Management

General Splinting Principles:

1. Always splint joints above and below a suspected fracture.
2. Pad bony prominences generously.
3. Avoid circumferential wrapping—risk of compartment syndrome.
4. Recheck neurovascular status post-splinting.

Common Splint Types:

1. Ulnar Gutter Splint: 4th/5th metacarpal fractures
2. Radial Gutter Splint: 2nd/3rd metacarpal fractures
3. Thumb Spica Splint: Scaphoid fracture, thumb injury
4. Volar Splint: Wrist sprain or distal radius fracture
5. Sugar Tong Splint: Distal radius or forearm fracture
6. Posterior Long Arm Splint: Elbow injury, olecranon fx
7. Posterior Short Leg Splint: Ankle sprain, metatarsal fx
8. Bulky Jones Splint: Severe ankle sprains or tibial shaft injury
9. Humeral Coaptation Splint: Humeral shaft fracture

Tips for Success:

1. Use cold water to slow plaster setting.
2. Mold the splint gently to avoid pressure points.
3. Elevate the limb post-application to reduce swelling.
4. Document time of application and neurovascular status.

When to Refer

Immediate Transfer:

1. Open fractures or compartment syndrome
2. Neurovascular compromise despite splint

3. Unstable fractures needing urgent surgery

Urgent Referral:

1. Displaced fractures needing reduction
2. Suspicion of missed joint dislocation
3. Persistent severe pain despite splint

Routine Follow-up:

1. Non-displaced fractures
2. Soft tissue injuries in stable patients
3. Review within 5–7 days for re-evaluation and definitive casting

Admission Orders

1. Admit to Rural Medicine – Limb Injury Requiring Immobilization
2. Diagnosis: [e.g., distal radius fracture]
3. Condition: Stable
4. Allergies: [Document here]

Orders:

1. Neurovascular checks q1h × 4, then q4h
2. Elevate limb
3. Pain management:
4. Acetaminophen 650 mg PO q6h
5. Morphine 2–4 mg IV q4h PRN
6. Keep splint dry and intact
7. Imaging: repeat X-ray if needed post-splint
8. Monitor for signs of compartment syndrome
9. Consult orthopedics if fracture alignment uncertain
10. Discharge Plan: Follow-up in fracture clinic or ortho in 5–7 days

Rural ER Pearls

1. Always document neurovascular status before and after splint application.
2. Avoid wrapping too tightly—especially in children and the elderly.
3. Pre-made aluminum foam splints can be useful when resources are limited.
4. Immobilize before transfer to reduce pain and prevent further injury.
5. Keep a splinting kit stocked and easily accessible in rural ERs.

CHAPTER 9
Orthopedic Splinting Techniques

Introduction

Proper splinting is a fundamental skill in rural emergency medicine. It serves to immobilize fractures, reduce pain and swelling, protect neurovascular structures, and prepare the patient for safe transfer. This chapter summarizes essential splinting techniques and their applications.

General Splinting Principles

1. Always assess and document neurovascular status before and after splinting.
2. Immobilize the joint above and below the fracture.
3. Use padding to prevent pressure sores, especially over bony prominences.
4. Do not circumferentially wrap wet plaster to avoid compartment syndrome.
5. Elevate and ice the splinted limb post-procedure.

Materials:

1. Plaster of Paris or fiberglass rolls
2. Webril (cotton padding)
3. Elastic wrap (ACE bandage)
4. Aluminum or prefabricated splints

Common Splints and Indications

1. Sugar Tong Splint

- For distal radius and ulnar fractures
- Prevents pronation/supination and flexion/extension

2. Posterior Long Arm Splint

- For elbow dislocations, proximal forearm fractures
- From upper arm to metacarpals, elbow at 90°

3. Volar Forearm Splint

- For wrist sprains, carpal fractures, soft tissue injuries

4. Thumb Spica Splint

- For scaphoid fractures, first metacarpal injuries

5. Ulnar Gutter Splint

- For 4th and 5th metacarpal fractures (Boxer's fracture)

6. Radial Gutter Splint

- For 2nd and 3rd metacarpal fractures

7. Posterior Short Leg Splint

- For ankle fractures, Achilles injuries, foot fractures

8. Stirrup Splint (U-shape)

- Stabilizes ankle for bimalleolar/trimalleolar fractures

9. Long Leg Splint

- For tibial shaft or knee injuries

10. Knee Immobilizer (prefab)

- For ligamentous injuries, patellar dislocations

Pediatric Considerations

1. Use lighter fiberglass material where possible.
2. Immobilize in functional position (e.g., wrist slight extension).
3. Avoid overtightening.
4. Reassess frequently in growing children due to swelling and circulation risk.

Post-Splinting Care

1. Recheck neurovascular status (cap refill, pulses, sensation, motor)
2. Provide sling, crutches, or walking boot as needed
3. Educate patient on signs of compartment syndrome (pain out of proportion, numbness, pallor, weakness)
4. Elevate and ice
5. Arrange follow-up with orthopedics or family physician

Rural ER Pearls

1. Practice splinting with simulation kits.
2. Prefabricated splints save time in high-volume ERs.
3. Document "neurovascular intact pre- and post-splint."
4. Be cautious with circumferential casting in swelling injuries.
5. Pad generously over pressure points (e.g., olecranon, malleoli).

CHAPTER 10
Orthopedic X-ray Interpretation Skills – Checklists and Lines for Each Joint

Introduction

Accurate interpretation of orthopedic X-rays is vital in the rural ER setting, where timely decisions must be made often without radiology support. This chapter outlines a systematic checklist approach and key anatomical lines for major joints to avoid missing subtle fractures or dislocations.

General Systematic Checklist for All Ortho Films

1. Patient and Image Details

- Confirm name, date, side, and correct projection views

2. Bones

- Trace cortex continuously
- Look for disruption, fracture lines, lucencies, sclerosis

3. Joints

- Check joint alignment and spacing
- Assess congruency and signs of dislocation or subluxation

4. Soft Tissues

- Look for effusion, fat pad signs, soft tissue swelling

5. Compare if Needed

- Consider comparison views (especially in pediatrics)

Shoulder X-ray – Key Views and Lines

1. Views: AP, Y-scapular, Axillary
2. Check anterior vs posterior dislocation (Y-view best)
3. Glenohumeral congruency
4. AC joint spacing
5. Look for Hill-Sachs or Bankart lesions in dislocations

Elbow X-ray – Pediatric and Adult

1. Views: AP and Lateral
2. Key line: **Anterior humeral line** (should intersect middle 1/3 of capitellum)
3. **Radiocapitellar line**: Radius should intersect capitellum on all views
4. Fat pad sign (posterior fat pad = occult fracture)
5. Supracondylar fractures common in kids

Wrist X-ray – Alignment and Carpal Arches

1. Views: PA, Lateral, Oblique
2. **Gilula's arcs** (3 smooth curves through carpal rows)
3. Scapholunate spacing < 3 mm
4. Look for distal radius fractures, scaphoid fracture
5. Assess radial inclination and volar tilt

Hand and Fingers

1. Check alignment and angulation of metacarpals and phalanges
2. Look for boxer's fracture (5th metacarpal neck)

3. Rotational deformities (evident when fingers not aligned on flexion)

Hip and Pelvis X-ray

1. Views: AP pelvis, frog-leg lateral
2. Shenton's line continuity
3. Assess femoral head position, sacroiliac joints, pubic symphysis
4. Subtle signs of femoral neck fracture: loss of trabecular continuity
5. Pediatric: Look for slipped capital femoral epiphysis (SCFE) and Perthes disease

Knee X-ray

1. Views: AP, lateral, sunrise (patellar)
2. Check joint spacing, tibial plateau alignment
3. Look for lipohemarthrosis (fat-fluid level) = intra-articular fracture
4. Patellar height (Insall-Salvati ratio)

Ankle and Foot X-ray

1. Views: AP, Mortise, Lateral
2. **Mortise view**: Should show even joint space around talus
3. Check fibular overlap and syndesmosis widening
4. Foot: Lisfranc alignment (medial base of 2nd metatarsal should align with medial cuneiform)

Cervical Spine X-ray (Trauma)

1. Views: Lateral, AP, Odontoid
2. Check for alignment: **Anterior, posterior vertebral lines, spinolaminar line**

3. Look for prevertebral soft tissue swelling
4. C1-C2 (odontoid): Ensure lateral masses aligned

DOCUMENTATION & MEDICOLEGAL

CHAPTER 11
Common Orthopedic Pitfalls and Documentation Errors

Introduction

Orthopedic complaints are common in rural emergency departments, and documentation errors or missed diagnoses can lead to serious consequences for patient safety and medicolegal risk. Awareness of common pitfalls helps improve outcomes, reduce unnecessary transfers, and protect clinicians in limited-resource settings.

Assessment

Risk Areas:

1. Missed fractures on X-ray (e.g., scaphoid, radial head, posterior shoulder)
2. Inadequate neurovascular documentation
3. Poor follow-up planning or unclear discharge instructions
4. Failure to reassess pain or function before discharge

Key Assessment Elements:

1. Mechanism of injury
2. Neurovascular exam before and after any procedure (motor, sensory, pulses, cap refill)
3. Range of motion, point tenderness, swelling
4. X-ray interpretation – include 2 views and note whether reviewed by radiology (if applicable)
5. Differential diagnosis (e.g., fracture, dislocation, sprain, infection)

Management

Common Pitfalls:

1. Failure to Document Neurovascular Status:

- Always document motor, sensation, pulses distal to injury
- Repeat after splinting or reduction

2. Discharging Suspected Scaphoid Fracture with "Normal" X-ray:

- Immobilize and arrange follow-up even if radiographs are unremarkable

3. Overlooking Compartment Syndrome or Open Fractures:

- Watch for escalating pain, tight compartments, decreased sensation or pulse

4. Inadequate Immobilization:

- Splint joints above and below
- Improper application can worsen injury

5. Not Providing Clear Follow-Up Plan:

- Who will reassess? When? Where?
- Include contact numbers and timing (e.g., ortho in 5–7 days)

6. Missed Associated Injuries:

- Look for secondary injuries (e.g., radial head fx with elbow dislocation)

When to Refer

Immediate Transfer:

1. Open fractures
2. Neurovascular compromise
3. Suspicion of compartment syndrome
4. Unstable joint dislocations

Urgent Referral:

1. Displaced fractures
2. Suspected septic arthritis or osteomyelitis
3. Inability to ambulate due to injury

Routine Follow-up:

1. Stable fractures or sprains with clear discharge instructions
2. Suspected scaphoid fractures
3. Reassessment of healing within 7–10 days

Admission Orders

1. Admit to Rural Medicine – Missed Fracture or Complicated Ortho Injury
2. Diagnosis: [e.g., missed midshaft humeral fracture with radial nerve palsy]
3. Condition: Stable
4. Allergies: [Document here]

Orders:

1. Vitals q4h, monitor for neurovascular changes
2. Immobilize limb
3. Repeat X-rays with appropriate views

Pain management:

1. Acetaminophen 650 mg PO q6h
2. Morphine 2–4 mg IV q4h PRN
3. Consult orthopedics
4. Document full neurovascular exam and reassess daily
5. Plan for transfer if surgical intervention needed
6. Discharge Plan: Follow-up in fracture clinic or ortho

Rural ER Pearls

1. Every ortho note should include: MOI, physical exam, neurovascular status (before/after), X-ray review, plan.
2. Use templates or macros if available to ensure nothing is missed.
3. Don't hesitate to splint and refer with a good note — even if diagnosis is uncertain.
4. A detailed discharge plan with return instructions prevents complications and complaints.
5. Ask patients to return sooner if worsening pain, numbness, or loss of function.

CHAPTER 12
Documentation & Medicolegal Pitfalls in Orthopedic Cases – High-Risk Situations in the Rural ER

Introduction

Orthopedic injuries are among the most commonly litigated cases in emergency medicine. In rural settings, where follow-up may be delayed and resources limited, proper documentation is essential to protect both patient safety and physician liability. This chapter highlights high-risk scenarios, key documentation strategies, and medicolegal traps to avoid.

High-Risk Orthopedic Presentations

1. Missed fractures (scaphoid, femoral neck, Lisfranc)
2. Delayed diagnosis of compartment syndrome
3. Open fractures not treated with early antibiotics
4. Dislocations reduced without post-reduction imaging
5. Failure to document neurovascular exam
6. Inadequate safety netting for discharge patients

Essential Documentation Elements

1. Mechanism of injury: Detail forces involved and timeline
2. Neurovascular exam: Must document before and after reduction/splinting
3. Imaging: Note views obtained and your interpretation
4. Management plan: Include pain control, splinting, antibiotics, tetanus
5. Reduction attempts: Note sedation, technique, and post-reduction assessment

6. Referral details: Who was contacted, when, and what advice was given
7. Discharge instructions: Red flags, follow-up plan, and activity restrictions
8. Patient consent and understanding: Especially for high-risk or non-transfer decisions

Common Medicolegal Pitfalls

1. No documentation of NV status = assumed not done
2. Handwritten notes not legible
3. Verbal referral not backed by written/faxed notes
4. Relying on verbal radiology read without reviewing images
5. Discharging patients without clear red flag advice
6. Using non-standard abbreviations or vague terms ("looks okay", "intact")

Practical Tips to Minimize Risk

1. Use checklists for fracture/dislocation documentation
2. Take photos of wounds or splints (if permitted by policy)
3. Clearly explain to patient the risk of delayed union, infection, re-injury
4. Record time-sensitive interventions (e.g., antibiotics within 1 hour)
5. Document who accepted transfer or gave advice – include time and name

Example Documentation Phrase

- "15-year-old male fell from skateboard, left wrist pain.
- Tender over anatomical snuffbox. X-ray negative for obvious fracture.

- NV exam: radial pulse 2+, cap refill <2s, sensation/motor intact.
- Thumb spica splint applied. Advised possible occult scaphoid fx – follow-up with ortho within 1 week. Return earlier for ↑ pain/swelling or numbness. Patient and parent understand and agree."

NEUROVASCULAR & COMPARTMENT

CHAPTER 13
Compartment Syndrome – Red Flag in Rural Orthopedic Emergencies

Introduction

Compartment syndrome is a surgical emergency resulting from increased pressure within a closed muscle compartment, leading to decreased perfusion, tissue ischemia, and potentially irreversible damage. Early recognition and immediate transfer for surgical decompression are critical, particularly in rural settings where access to orthopedic care may be delayed.

Assessment

Classic Causes:

1. Long bone fractures (especially tibia)
2. Crush injuries or prolonged limb compression
3. Reperfusion after ischemia
4. Tight casts or splints
5. Burns or high-pressure injection injuries

The 5 P's of Compartment Syndrome:

1. Pain out of proportion (earliest and most sensitive sign)
2. Paresthesia (tingling or numbness)
3. Pallor (late finding)
4. Paralysis (late finding)
5. Pulselessness (very late and unreliable)

Additional Clinical Features:

1. Pain with passive stretch of muscles in compartment
2. Tense, swollen, shiny skin over compartment

3. Decreased sensation or motor strength
4. Compartment pressure measurement (if available): >30 mmHg is suggestive of compartment syndrome

Management

DO NOT delay:

1. Remove any constrictive dressings, casts, or splints immediately
2. Elevate the limb to heart level (not above)
3. Administer IV fluids for rhabdomyolysis risk
4. Provide analgesia and oxygen

Urgent Transfer Protocol:

1. Immediate transfer to surgical center with orthopedic capability
2. Document time of assessment and deterioration
3. Monitor urine output if rhabdomyolysis suspected
4. Consider IV bicarbonate if metabolic acidosis present
5. Do not wait for imaging. Diagnosis is clinical.

When to Refer

Immediate Transfer:

1. Any suspicion of compartment syndrome
2. Pain out of proportion + passive stretch pain or neurologic findings
3. Trauma with high risk of crush or bleeding into compartment
4. Do not attempt fasciotomy in rural settings unless trained and equipped

Admission Orders

1. Admit to Rural Medicine – Suspected Compartment Syndrome (Stabilization Only)
2. Diagnosis: Suspected acute compartment syndrome, [e.g., left forearm]
3. Condition: Critical
4. Allergies: [Document here]

Orders:

1. Vitals q1h, monitor limb neurovascular status
2. Remove splints/dressings
3. IV NS bolus 1–2 L, then maintenance at 100 mL/h
4. Monitor urine output q2h, consider Foley catheter
5. Pain control:
6. Morphine 2–4 mg IV q4h PRN
7. Labs:
8. CBC, CK, Cr, Lytes, Lactate, ABG
9. Call receiving hospital – orthopedic transfer
10. Do not delay transfer for imaging or labs if diagnosis is clear

Rural ER Pearls

1. Pain out of proportion is the most important early sign.
2. Delayed diagnosis can lead to permanent nerve/muscle damage or amputation.
3. Don't be reassured by normal pulses — compartment syndrome can occur with intact vasculature.
4. Always reassess patients with limb trauma within hours.
5. Fasciotomy must be done by an experienced surgeon; initiate transfer immediately if suspected.

CHAPTER 14
Neurovascular Compromise in Limb Injuries

Introduction

Neurovascular compromise is a critical concern in limb injuries. Delayed diagnosis can lead to irreversible damage, limb loss, or death. Rural providers must recognize subtle signs and initiate urgent stabilization and transfer for definitive care. This chapter outlines recognition, key assessments, and emergency management of suspected neurovascular injuries in the rural emergency department.

Assessment

Mechanisms of Concern:

1. High-energy trauma (e.g., motor vehicle collisions, falls)
2. Fractures near major vessels (supracondylar, femoral, pelvic, knee dislocations)
3. Crush injuries
4. Penetrating injuries (e.g., stab, gunshot)

Key Components of the Neurovascular Exam:

1. Motor: Test distal muscle groups (e.g., wrist/finger extension, foot dorsiflexion)
2. Sensation: Light touch, pinprick in dermatomes
3. Pulses: Palpable? Doppler?
4. Capillary Refill: Normal <2 seconds
5. Skin Temperature and Colour

5 P's of Limb Threat:

1. Pain (disproportionate to injury)
2. Paresthesia
3. Pallor

4. Paralysis
5. Pulselessness (late and unreliable)

Document findings clearly on initial and serial exams

Management

Immediate Actions:

1. Expose and inspect the limb
2. Remove any constrictive devices (e.g., splints, bandages)
3. Reposition dislocations if pulseless limb and trained (e.g., knee dislocation with absent DP pulse)
4. Apply gentle splinting and elevate to heart level
5. IV fluids if shock is suspected
6. Pain management with IV analgesia

Doppler Exam (if available):

1. Assess for diminished or absent flow
2. Document location of last palpable pulse

Prepare for Urgent Transfer:

1. Contact receiving center early
2. Mark pulse sites
3. Elevate limb and immobilize
4. Do NOT delay transfer for imaging in suspected arterial injury

When to Refer

Immediate Transfer:

1. Absent or diminished pulses in injured limb
2. New or worsening motor or sensory deficit
3. Expanding hematoma, bruit, thrill over injury
4. Suspected arterial laceration or thrombosis

5. Dislocations with vascular involvement (e.g., knee dislocation)

Urgent Referral:

1. Suspected nerve injuries (e.g., radial, peroneal palsy)
2. Progressive swelling with evolving deficits

Routine Follow-Up:

1. Minor contusions with normal neurovascular exam
2. Documented nerve deficits with stable fracture (orthopedic referral within days)

Admission Orders

1. Admit to Rural Medicine – Suspected Neurovascular Compromise (Stabilization Phase)
2. Diagnosis: [e.g., right knee dislocation with absent DP pulse]
3. Condition: Critical
4. Allergies: [Document here]

Orders:

1. Vitals q1h, limb NV status q1h
2. Elevate and splint injured limb
3. IV NS 100 mL/h
4. Morphine 2–4 mg IV q4h PRN
5. CBC, Cr, Lytes, CK, INR/PTT, crossmatch
6. Document full NV exam and repeat hourly
7. Doppler if available
8. Urgent surgical consultation and transfer arrangements
9. NPO in anticipation of surgery

Rural ER Pearls

1. Document the **neurovascular status before and after** any manipulation or splinting.
2. If pulse is absent but Doppler flow is present, treat as urgent.
3. Use serial exams to catch evolving deficits.
4. A pulseless limb is a surgical emergency — act fast and communicate clearly.
5. Communicate time of injury and last known normal exam when referring.

INFECTION & INFLAMMATORY JOINT

CHAPTER 15
Antibiotic and Tetanus Protocols in Orthopedic Injuries – Open Fractures, Bites, and Rust Wounds

Introduction

Prompt antibiotic and tetanus prophylaxis is essential in managing orthopedic injuries with a risk of infection. This is particularly critical in rural emergency settings, where delays in definitive surgical care may increase the risk of complications. This chapter outlines evidence-based protocols for common high-risk scenarios: open fractures, animal/human bites, and puncture wounds from contaminated objects (e.g., nails, rusty metal).

Open Fractures – Antibiotic Protocol

1. Start antibiotics as soon as possible (ideally within 1 hour of presentation).
2. Type I/II: Cefazolin 1–2 g IV q8h (Clindamycin if allergic)
3. Type III or heavily contaminated: Add Gentamicin + Metronidazole for anaerobic coverage
4. Do not delay antibiotics for X-ray or ortho consultation
5. Document time of administration
6. Update tetanus as needed

Animal and Human Bites – Protocol

1. High risk for polymicrobial infection (aerobes + anaerobes)
2. Antibiotic of choice: Amoxicillin-clavulanate 875/125 mg PO BID for 5–7 days

3. If allergic: Doxycycline + Metronidazole (adults) or Clindamycin + TMP-SMX
4. Copious irrigation and wound exploration
5. Avoid closure unless on face or for cosmetic need
6. Ensure tetanus vaccination up to date

Rusty Nails / Puncture Wounds – Protocol

Treat as contaminated wound – high risk for Clostridium tetani and Pseudomonas

Tetanus prophylaxis:

1. Clean wound, tetanus vaccine >10 yrs ago → Give Td booster
2. Dirty wound, vaccine >5 yrs ago or uncertain → Give Td + TIG (tetanus immune globulin)

Antibiotics:

1. For plantar punctures (e.g., through shoe): Ciprofloxacin for Pseudomonas coverage
2. Otherwise: Cephalexin or Clindamycin based on severity

Documentation Pearls

1. Record antibiotic name, dose, route, and time given
2. Specify tetanus vaccine status and action taken
3. Note wound classification (e.g., open fracture type)
4. Include reason for antibiotic choice in complex cases

CHAPTER 16
Approach to the Swollen Joint – Monoarthritis

Introduction

A single swollen joint (monoarthritis) can be a diagnostic challenge in the rural emergency department. Causes range from benign trauma to urgent conditions such as septic arthritis or hemarthrosis. Prompt evaluation and treatment are essential to prevent joint damage, especially when access to imaging or aspiration is limited.

Assessment

History:

1. Onset: acute vs gradual
2. Trauma history (minor or major)
3. Associated fever, chills, malaise
4. Prior joint disease (e.g., gout, OA, RA)
5. Risk factors: immunosuppression, recent surgery, STI exposure

Physical Exam:

1. Inspect for erythema, swelling, effusion
2. Palpate for warmth, tenderness
3. Assess active/passive ROM
4. Evaluate adjacent joints and look for systemic signs

Common Causes:

1. Septic arthritis (urgent!)
2. Gout or pseudogout
3. Trauma with hemarthrosis

4. Osteoarthritis flare
5. Reactive arthritis
6. Lyme disease or viral arthritis

Investigations:

1. Joint aspiration (if trained): send for WBC, Gram stain, culture, crystals
2. CBC, ESR, CRP
3. Uric acid level (not diagnostic during acute flare)
4. Blood cultures if febrile
5. X-ray to assess for fracture, effusion, or chondrocalcinosis

Management

Initial ED Management:

1. Immobilize joint and provide analgesia
2. If septic arthritis suspected:
3. Empiric IV antibiotics (e.g., ceftriaxone or vancomycin)
4. Arrange urgent transfer for washout

If gout suspected:

1. NSAIDs (e.g., naproxen 500 mg PO BID) or colchicine
2. Consider intra-articular steroids if no infection risk
3. Avoid aspiration unless sterile technique and local experience allow

Supportive Measures:

1. Ice, elevation
2. Crutches or sling if weight-bearing joint involved
3. Hydration and rest

When to Refer

Immediate Transfer:

1. Suspected septic arthritis (esp. hip or shoulder)
2. Hemarthrosis with ongoing bleeding
3. Monoarthritis with systemic signs (fever, tachycardia)

Urgent Referral:

1. Gout not responding to therapy
2. Suspicion of autoimmune disease
3. Joint effusion needing diagnostic aspiration

Routine Follow-up:

1. Gout, pseudogout with good symptom control
2. Osteoarthritis flare without red flags
3. Minor trauma with no fracture on X-ray

Admission Orders

1. Admit to Rural Medicine – Suspected Septic Arthritis
2. Diagnosis: [e.g., monoarthritis – R knee, possible septic]
3. Condition: Stable
4. Allergies: [Document here]

Orders:

1. Vitals q4h, monitor for fever
2. IV fluids: NS at 75 mL/h
3. Empiric antibiotics:
4. Ceftriaxone 2 g IV q24h ± vancomycin 15 mg/kg IV q12h
5. CBC, ESR, CRP daily

6. Joint aspiration if able – send for culture, Gram stain, crystals
7. X-ray of affected joint
8. Pain management:
9. Acetaminophen 650 mg PO q6h
10. Morphine 2–4 mg IV q4h PRN
11. Rheumatology consult if autoimmune disease suspected
12. Discharge Plan: Based on culture results and improvement

Rural ER Pearls

1. Septic arthritis is a joint-threatening emergency—don't miss it.
2. Intra-articular steroid injection is contraindicated until infection ruled out.
3. Knee is the most commonly affected joint.
4. Crystal identification under polarized light is diagnostic for gout/pseudogout.
5. Joint aspiration is both diagnostic and therapeutic—know when to refer if unable to perform.

CHAPTER 17
Necrotizing Fasciitis of Limbs

Introduction

Necrotizing fasciitis is a rapidly progressive, life-threatening soft tissue infection that involves the fascia and subcutaneous tissues. It can affect any part of the body but is particularly devastating in the limbs. Prompt recognition and surgical intervention are essential to reduce morbidity and mortality. In rural emergency settings, early suspicion, initiation of broad-spectrum antibiotics, and urgent transfer for surgical management are critical.

Assessment

History:

1. Rapid onset limb pain, often out of proportion to physical findings
2. Recent trauma, surgery, injection, or skin breach
3. Underlying conditions: diabetes, immunosuppression, peripheral vascular disease
4. Systemic symptoms: fever, malaise, confusion

Physical Exam:

1. Erythema, swelling, and tenderness over affected area
2. Pain out of proportion to visible skin changes
3. Skin changes: violaceous discoloration, bullae, necrosis
4. Crepitus (gas in tissue) in some cases
5. Signs of septic shock: hypotension, tachycardia, altered mental status

Imaging:

1. Primarily a clinical diagnosis—do not delay treatment for imaging
2. X-ray: may show gas in soft tissues
3. CT or MRI: can delineate fascial involvement if available without delaying surgery

Laboratory Findings:

1. Leukocytosis, elevated CRP
2. Metabolic acidosis, elevated lactate
3. LRINEC (Laboratory Risk Indicator for Necrotizing Fasciitis) score may aid diagnosis but is not definitive

Management

Immediate Actions:

1. Call surgical team immediately—this is a surgical emergency
2. Start broad-spectrum IV antibiotics:
3. Piperacillin-tazobactam 4.5 g IV q6h + clindamycin 900 mg IV q8h + vancomycin (weight-based dosing)
4. Aggressive IV fluid resuscitation
5. Pain control with opioids if needed
6. Oxygen supplementation as required

Do Not:

1. Delay surgical consultation for imaging unless absolutely necessary
2. Attempt bedside incision/drainage without surgical backup—this condition requires wide debridement

When to Refer

Immediate Transfer:

1. All suspected cases require urgent transfer to a facility with surgical capability
2. Continue resuscitation and antibiotics during transfer

Admission Orders

1. Admit to Rural Medicine – Necrotizing Fasciitis (Pre-Transfer Management)
2. Diagnosis: Suspected necrotizing fasciitis of limb
3. Condition: Critical
4. Allergies: [Document here]

Orders:

1. Vitals q15–30min
2. Oxygen via nasal cannula or mask to maintain SpO$_2$ >94%
3. IV fluids: normal saline boluses as needed
4. IV antibiotics:
5. Piperacillin-tazobactam 4.5 g IV q6h
6. Clindamycin 900 mg IV q8h
7. Vancomycin IV (dose per weight and renal function)
8. Analgesia: Morphine 2–5 mg IV q1h PRN
9. Monitor urine output with catheter
10. Prepare patient for transfer with documentation and labs

Rural ER Pearls

1. Pain out of proportion to exam is a red flag—consider necrotizing fasciitis early
2. Early surgical debridement is the most important life-saving step

3. Use broad-spectrum antibiotics covering gram-positive, gram-negative, and anaerobes
4. Continue aggressive resuscitation during transfer

CHAPTER 18
Osteomyelitis in Open Injuries or Diabetics – Rural Emergency Approach

Introduction

Osteomyelitis is a serious bone infection that may present acutely or subacutely, particularly in patients with open fractures, puncture wounds, or diabetic foot ulcers. Rural emergency physicians must have a high index of suspicion, initiate early antibiotics, and plan for timely referral to prevent chronic infection or systemic complications.

Assessment

Populations at Risk:

1. Open fractures or penetrating trauma
2. Diabetic foot infections, especially with ulcers over bony prominences
3. Immunosuppressed patients
4. Chronic wounds or surgical sites
5. Pediatric patients with localized bone pain and fever

Clinical Features:

1. Localized bone pain, swelling, warmth, erythema
2. Fever may be absent, especially in chronic or diabetic cases
3. Draining sinus tract or exposed bone
4. Elevated CRP, ESR, WBC
5. Positive probe-to-bone test in diabetic foot ulcer (sensitive for osteomyelitis)

Imaging:

1. Plain X-ray: May be normal early; look for periosteal elevation or lytic lesions later
2. MRI (if available) is the gold standard for early detection
3. Bone scan or nuclear imaging if MRI not accessible

Management

Early empiric IV antibiotics based on source:

1. Diabetic foot: Pip-Tazo 3.375 g IV q6h OR Ceftriaxone + Metronidazole
2. Open trauma: Cefazolin 2 g IV q8h + Gentamicin 5 mg/kg IV once
3. Consider MRSA coverage (Vancomycin) in chronic or healthcare-associated cases

Additional Measures:

1. Debride necrotic tissue
2. Wound care with sterile saline dressings
3. Offload pressure from affected limb
4. Ensure glycemic control in diabetic patients
5. NPO if transfer likely for surgical debridement

When to Refer

Urgent Transfer:

1. Suspected osteomyelitis with systemic symptoms or rapidly worsening condition
2. Exposed bone or necrotic tissue
3. Inadequate local imaging or wound care capacity
4. Lack of IV antibiotic coverage in rural setting

Outpatient Referral:

1. Stable patients with subacute symptoms
2. Able to arrange prompt follow-up for MRI and infectious disease or ortho consult

Document:

1. Onset and duration of symptoms
2. Risk factors (e.g., diabetes, trauma)
3. Exam findings and any imaging performed

Admission Orders

1. Admit to Rural Medicine – Suspected Osteomyelitis
2. Diagnosis: [e.g., Left diabetic foot ulcer with exposed bone – likely osteomyelitis]
3. Condition: Stable or Critical (specify)
4. Allergies: [Document here]

Orders:

1. Vitals q4h
2. IV NS at 100 mL/h
3. Pip-Tazo 3.375 g IV q6h OR Ceftriaxone 2 g IV + Metronidazole 500 mg IV q8h
4. CBC, Cr, Lytes, ESR, CRP, blood cultures ×2
5. Wound culture from deep tissue if possible
6. Wound care: NS irrigation and sterile dressing BID
7. Bed rest and offload affected foot
8. Accuchecks q6h and manage blood glucose
9. Arrange urgent transfer or follow-up for MRI and surgical consult

Rural ER Pearls

1. Always probe foot ulcers to assess for bone exposure.
2. Chronic wounds with new pain/swelling should raise concern for osteomyelitis.
3. Do not rely on normal early X-rays to exclude diagnosis.
4. Avoid prolonged oral antibiotics without imaging confirmation or specialist input.
5. Glycemic control is essential in diabetic wound healing.

CHAPTER 19
Septic Joint – Rural Approach and Urgent Management

Introduction

Septic arthritis is a limb- and life-threatening condition requiring early recognition, joint aspiration, and intravenous antibiotics. Delay in diagnosis can lead to rapid joint destruction, especially in weight-bearing joints like the hip or knee. This chapter outlines a practical rural emergency approach to this critical diagnosis.

Assessment

Clinical Features:

1. Acute monoarthritis (commonly knee > hip > shoulder)
2. Joint pain, swelling, warmth, redness
3. Fever or systemic symptoms (may be absent in elderly or immunocompromised)
4. Painful passive and active ROM
5. Inability to bear weight

Risk Factors:

1. Recent joint surgery or trauma
2. Prosthetic joint
3. Immunosuppression or diabetes
4. IV drug use
5. Pre-existing joint disease (e.g., RA, gout)

Differential Diagnosis:

1. Gout or pseudogout
2. Reactive arthritis

3. Hemarthrosis
4. Trauma or fracture

Labs:

1. CBC, ESR, CRP (often elevated)
2. Blood cultures ×2
3. Uric acid (to rule out gout)
4. Consider STI screening in young adults

Joint Aspiration:

1. Send fluid for:
2. Gram stain and culture
3. Cell count with differential (>50,000 WBC highly suggestive)
4. Crystals
5. Do NOT inject steroids before ruling out infection

Management

Do not delay treatment for aspiration if septic arthritis is strongly suspected.

Empiric IV Antibiotics:

1. Native Joint: Ceftriaxone 2 g IV daily
2. Add Vancomycin 15 mg/kg IV q12h if concern for MRSA or prosthetic joint
3. Consider coverage for gonorrhea in sexually active young adults

Additional Measures:

1. Immobilize the joint
2. Elevate limb
3. IV fluids and analgesia
4. NPO if surgery anticipated

    5. Avoid NSAIDs in septic joint until infection excluded

When to Refer

Urgent Transfer:

1. Any suspected septic joint, especially hip
2. Inability to aspirate joint or no improvement within hours
3. Prosthetic joints
4. Systemic signs of sepsis
5. Rapid joint swelling or deterioration

Local follow-up only if:

1. Low suspicion after aspiration
2. Crystals identified without infection signs
3. Stable vital signs and no systemic illness

Admission Orders

1. Admit to Rural Medicine – Suspected Septic Arthritis
2. Diagnosis: [e.g., Septic arthritis – right knee]
3. Condition: Critical
4. Allergies: [Document here]

Orders:

1. Vitals q1h, monitor for sepsis
2. IV NS at 100 mL/h
3. Ceftriaxone 2 g IV q24h
4. Add Vancomycin 15 mg/kg IV q12h if prosthetic or MRSA risk
5. Joint aspiration if trained
6. Send for gram stain, culture, cell count, crystals
7. Blood cultures ×2
8. CBC, Cr, Lytes, CRP, ESR, uric acid

9. Immobilize joint with splint
10. Acetaminophen 650 mg PO q6h PRN
11. Call orthopedic referral center and arrange urgent transfer

Rural ER Pearls

1. Septic arthritis may lack fever, especially in elderly or immunocompromised.
2. Start antibiotics only after blood cultures and aspiration unless critically ill.
3. Hip septic arthritis can present with vague groin pain — maintain a high index of suspicion.
4. Do not delay transfer to aspirate if skill or imaging is unavailable.
5. Always rule out STI-related septic arthritis in young adults (especially gonococcal).

PEDIATRICS & CHILD PROTECTION

CHAPTER 20
Non-Accidental Injury in Children –
Fractures Suggestive of Abuse

Introduction

Recognizing non-accidental trauma (NAT) is a critical responsibility for rural emergency physicians. Some fractures are highly suggestive of child abuse, particularly in infants and non-ambulatory children. Timely identification, documentation, and reporting can save lives and prevent further harm.

Assessment

History:

1. Inconsistent history or delay in seeking care
2. Mechanism not plausible for developmental age
3. History changes with retelling or differs between caregivers
4. Previous ED visits or known child protection involvement

Physical Exam:

1. Full head-to-toe examination, including back and genitalia
2. Bruising in unusual locations (e.g., torso, ears, neck)
3. Multiple fractures in various healing stages
4. Burns, bite marks, or signs of neglect

Fractures Suspicious for Abuse:

1. Classic metaphyseal lesions (CML) or "bucket handle" fractures

2. Posterior rib fractures (esp. in infants)
3. Scapular fractures
4. Spinous process or sternal fractures
5. Complex skull fractures
6. Femur fractures in non-ambulatory children
7. Multiple fractures in different stages of healing

Investigations:

1. X-rays of affected area
2. Skeletal survey (especially under age 2)
3. Head CT if any signs of head trauma
4. Labs: coagulation profile to rule out bleeding disorder
5. Consider retinal exam for suspected head injury (by ophthalmology)

Management

Initial ED Management:

1. Provide analgesia and stabilize injuries
2. Avoid accusatory language with caregivers
3. Ensure child safety while investigation proceeds
4. Involve social worker or child protection services immediately

Do Not:

1. Delay reporting while awaiting full workup
2. Confront caregivers without support
3. Discharge the child without documenting plan

Documentation:

1. Record detailed injury description, caregiver explanations
2. Note inconsistencies, affect, and behaviors

3. Use objective language (e.g., "caregiver reports...", "child observed to...")

When to Refer

Immediate Referral:

1. All suspected NAT must be reported to child protection services
2. Involve pediatrician or hospital with pediatric expertise
3. If unstable, transfer to tertiary center for full evaluation

Urgent (within 1–3 days):

1. Follow-up for skeletal survey, specialist input
2. Coordination with multidisciplinary team

Routine Follow-up:

1. Not applicable; every case of suspected abuse needs clear documentation and follow-up

Admission Orders

1. Admit to Rural Medicine – Suspected Non-Accidental Trauma
2. Diagnosis: [e.g., suspected rib fractures due to abuse]
3. Condition: Stable
4. Allergies: [Document here]

Orders:

1. Vitals q4h, continuous monitoring if <1 year
2. Pain management:
3. Acetaminophen 15 mg/kg PO q6h
4. Morphine 0.1 mg/kg IV q4h PRN
5. Skeletal survey (if under 2 years)
6. Head CT if head injury suspected

7. Labs: CBC, INR/PTT, LFTs
8. Notify child protection services and document time/contact person
9. Social work consult
10. Ophthalmology consult for retinal hemorrhage if head trauma
11. NPO if surgery is anticipated
12. Discharge Plan: Pending multidisciplinary decision

Rural ER Pearls

1. Posterior rib fractures, metaphyseal lesions, and long bone fractures in infants are red flags.
2. Skeletal survey is essential in children <2 years with suspicious injuries.
3. Any delay in seeking care or inconsistent history warrants deeper investigation.
4. Reporting suspected abuse is a legal and ethical obligation—no confirmation required.
5. Early multidisciplinary involvement improves outcomes and protects the child.

CHAPTER 21
Nursemaid's Elbow (Radial Head Subluxation)

Introduction

Nursemaid's elbow, or radial head subluxation, is a common pediatric injury, usually seen in children aged 1–5 years. It occurs when axial traction is applied to the extended and pronated forearm, causing the annular ligament to slip over the radial head. Prompt recognition and reduction in the rural emergency setting can restore function immediately, avoiding unnecessary imaging or prolonged discomfort.

Assessment

History:

1. Mechanism: sudden pulling on the arm (lifting, swinging, yanking)
2. Immediate pain and refusal to use the arm
3. Arm often held close to body with elbow slightly flexed and forearm pronated
4. No significant swelling or bruising

Physical Exam:

1. Child guards the affected arm and resists movement
2. No deformity, significant swelling, or bruising
3. Tenderness over radial head possible but minimal
4. Full neurovascular function

Imaging:

1. Usually not required if presentation is classic

2. Obtain X-ray only if significant swelling, deformity, or suspicion of fracture

Management

Reduction Techniques:

1. Supination–Flexion Method:

- Support elbow, supinate forearm, then flex elbow while applying gentle pressure over radial head

2. Hyperpronation Method:

- Support elbow, hyperpronate forearm while stabilizing radial head
- A palpable or audible click may be felt during successful reduction
- Child usually resumes arm use within minutes

3. Post-Reduction:

- Observe for 10–15 minutes to ensure return of function
- No splinting required if child regains full use of arm
- Educate caregivers to avoid traction injuries

When to Refer

Immediate Referral:

1. Failed reduction attempts
2. Suspicion of fracture or dislocation
3. Persistent pain or refusal to use arm after 15–30 minutes post-reduction

---

DR. MOHAMED ELGENDY, LMCC, CCFP, CANADA

Admission Orders

1. Usually not required for isolated nursemaid's elbow if successfully reduced.
2. If admitted for observation due to other concerns:
3. Diagnosis: Nursemaid's elbow – post-reduction observation
4. Condition: Stable
5. Allergies: [Document here]

Orders:

1. Vitals q4h
2. Analgesia:
3. Acetaminophen 15 mg/kg PO q6h PRN
4. Ibuprofen 10 mg/kg PO q6h PRN
5. Neurovascular checks q4h
6. Discharge once child uses arm normally

Rural ER Pearls

1. Hyperpronation method has slightly higher first-attempt success rate
2. Always reassure both child and caregivers before reduction
3. Avoid unnecessary imaging in classic presentations
4. Educate parents on prevention—avoid pulling or swinging child by the hands/arms

80

CHAPTER 22
Orthopedic Emergencies in Children – Growth Plate Injuries and Non-Accidental Trauma

Introduction

Pediatric orthopedic emergencies require a high index of suspicion, especially in rural settings. Growth plate (physeal) injuries can lead to long-term growth disturbances if missed or mistreated. Additionally, non-accidental trauma (NAT) must be carefully assessed in infants and young children presenting with fractures. This chapter outlines key assessment and management strategies for both.

Assessment of Growth Plate Injuries

1. Use the Salter-Harris classification (Types I–V) to describe physeal injuries.
2. Most common in distal radius, distal tibia, and fingers.
3. Often subtle on X-ray — compare with the contralateral limb if in doubt.
4. Type I and V may not be visible on initial imaging.
5. Mechanism of injury may be low-impact (e.g., fall from standing).

Clinical Features:

1. Localized tenderness over the growth plate
2. Swelling, decreased ROM
3. Pain with weight-bearing or manipulation
4. May appear "normal" on X-ray

81

Imaging:

1. Plain X-ray (AP and lateral) of joint above and below
2. Consider repeat imaging or referral if high suspicion but normal initial film

Assessment of Non-Accidental Trauma (NAT)

Always consider NAT in:

1. Infants with any fracture
2. Toddlers with spiral fractures of long bones without a clear mechanism
3. Multiple fractures at various stages of healing
4. Posterior rib fractures, metaphyseal corner fractures
5. Delay in seeking care or inconsistent history

Red Flags:

1. Injuries not consistent with developmental stage
2. Caregiver reports low-impact trauma for significant injury
3. Signs of neglect or other physical abuse (burns, bruises)

Mandatory steps:

1. Document exact history, mechanism, and quotes from caregiver
2. Notify child protection services if any suspicion
3. Involve social work or pediatrician if available

Management

Growth Plate Injuries:

1. Immobilization with splint or cast
2. Avoid manipulation in field if unstable fracture
3. Type I and II: Often managed conservatively

4. Type III–V: Require urgent ortho referral due to risk of joint surface or growth disturbance

NAT Suspicions:

1. Ensure child safety first
2. Document all findings in neutral language
3. Do not discharge until child protection team is involved
4. Avoid accusations — focus on objective findings

When to Refer

Urgent Ortho Referral:

1. Suspected Salter-Harris III–V injuries
2. Displaced fractures involving the physis
3. Suspicion of compartment syndrome or vascular compromise
4. Any toddler fracture if ambulation impaired

Urgent Child Protection Referral:

1. Any suspected non-accidental trauma
2. Multiple fractures, rib fractures, or skull fracture without clear trauma
3. Inconsistent stories or delayed presentation

Admission Orders (Sample – Suspected NAT)

1. Admit to Pediatrics – Suspected Non-Accidental Injury
2. Diagnosis: [e.g., Suspected NAT – spiral humerus fracture in 6-month-old]
3. Condition: Stable
4. Allergies: [Document here]

Orders:

1. Vitals q4h
2. CBC, Cr, LFTs, Coags
3. Skeletal survey
4. Social work consult
5. Notify Child Protection Services
6. Immobilize limb with appropriate splint
7. Pain management: Acetaminophen or ibuprofen PRN
8. Document detailed history and findings

Rural ER Pearls

1. Always compare both limbs when assessing for physeal injuries.
2. Growth plate injuries may present without visible fractures.
3. Maintain a low threshold for referral in pediatric fractures.
4. Trust your clinical intuition when history doesn't match the injury.
5. Documentation is critical in suspected child abuse cases — quote caregivers directly and include timeline inconsistencies.

CHAPTER 23
Pediatric Fractures

Introduction

Pediatric fractures are common in rural emergency settings. Due to growth plate involvement and unique remodeling potential in children, fracture management differs significantly from adults. Early recognition, proper splinting, and referral to pediatric orthopedic services are essential to avoid long-term complications.

Assessment

History:

1. Mechanism: fall, sports, abuse suspicion (non-ambulatory child with fracture)
2. Timing and progression of symptoms
3. Dominant hand, previous injuries

Physical Exam:

1. Inspect for deformity, swelling, bruising
2. Palpate the entire limb
3. Assess for tenderness over growth plates (physis)
4. Neurovascular exam (cap refill, pulses, sensation, movement)

Imaging:

1. Always include joint above and below
2. Pediatric bones show more growth plates and variable ossification centers
3. Use comparison views in uncertain cases (e.g., elbow injuries)
4. Salter-Harris classification for growth plate injuries

Management

Initial ED Management:

1. Immobilize with well-padded splint (sugar tong, posterior slab, etc.)
2. Analgesia: acetaminophen, ibuprofen, oral morphine if needed
3. Elevation and ice
4. Avoid circumferential casting in the ED to prevent compartment syndrome

Common Fractures and Pearls:

1. Buckle (torus) fracture: stable, treat with splinting
2. Greenstick fracture: may require reduction
3. Supracondylar humerus fracture: beware of brachial artery and median nerve injury
4. Forearm fractures: maintain alignment and rotation
5. Salter-Harris Type I/II: usually managed non-operatively
6. Type III/IV: require ortho referral

Do Not:

1. Miss signs of abuse: inconsistent history, multiple fractures in different stages
2. Delay referral for displaced or physeal injuries
3. Apply tight casts in ED

When to Refer

Immediate Transfer:

1. Open fractures
2. Neurovascular compromise
3. Displaced supracondylar humerus fracture

4. Suspected abuse

Urgent Referral (within 1–3 days):

1. Displaced or angulated fractures
2. Salter-Harris III/IV injuries
3. Non-urgent open fracture after initial care

Routine Follow-up:

1. Buckle fractures
2. Undisplaced fractures in stable patients
3. Minor greenstick or toddler's fractures with good alignment

Admission Orders

1. Admit to Rural Medicine – Pediatric Fracture
2. Diagnosis: [e.g., supracondylar humerus fracture]
3. Condition: Stable
4. Allergies: [Document here]

Orders:

1. Vitals q4h, neurovascular checks q2h x 24h
2. Analgesia:
3. Acetaminophen 15 mg/kg PO q6h
4. Ibuprofen 10 mg/kg PO q8h
5. Morphine 0.1 mg/kg IV q4h PRN
6. Immobilization: Posterior slab or sugar tong splint
7. NPO if surgery is anticipated
8. Labs: CBC, coagulation profile if OR planned
9. Imaging: X-ray with ortho review
10. Referral: Pediatric orthopedic service
11. Discharge Plan: Stable, splinted, follow-up arranged

Rural ER Pearls

1. Children remodel fractures well—acceptable angulation is age-dependent.
2. Always examine and document neurovascular status before and after splinting.
3. Suspect non-accidental trauma in infants or odd patterns (e.g., spiral femur fractures).
4. Salter-Harris classification is crucial for growth plate injuries.
5. Involve parents early and clearly explain the need for specialist follow-up.

CHAPTER 24
Septic Joint vs Transient Synovitis in Children – Rural Emergency Approach

Introduction

Limp or refusal to bear weight in children is a common yet potentially serious presentation in rural emergency settings. The key diagnostic dilemma often lies in differentiating between benign **transient synovitis** and limb-threatening **septic arthritis**. Prompt recognition of red flags, appropriate investigations, and timely transfer are crucial to avoid permanent joint damage.

Assessment

History:

1. Age: Transient synovitis most common in 3–8 years; septic arthritis can occur at any age
2. Onset: Sudden onset of limp vs gradual
3. Fever: Common in septic arthritis, absent or low-grade in transient synovitis
4. Recent viral illness: Often precedes transient synovitis
5. Weight-bearing: Inability suggests septic joint
6. Pain: Night pain or rest pain more concerning

Physical Exam:

1. Vital signs: Especially temperature and heart rate
2. Limb position: Hip typically held in flexion, abduction, and external rotation in septic arthritis
3. ROM: Pain with passive movement suggests joint involvement
4. Gait: Antalgic vs refusal to walk
5. Joint swelling, warmth, erythema

Kocher Criteria (Hip):

1. Non–weight bearing on affected side
2. ESR >40 mm/hr
3. Fever >38.5°C
4. WBC >12,000/mm³
5. ≥3 criteria: high likelihood of septic arthritis

Investigations:

1. CBC, CRP, ESR
2. Blood cultures
3. Ultrasound of joint (to detect effusion)
4. X-ray to rule out fracture or Perthes
5. Joint aspiration (if feasible) for cell count, Gram stain, culture

Management

If Septic Arthritis Suspected:

1. NPO
2. IV antibiotics:
3. Cefazolin or ceftriaxone empirically
4. Add vancomycin if MRSA risk
5. Analgesia: acetaminophen, ibuprofen, morphine
6. Urgent transfer to tertiary care for joint aspiration and possible washout

If Transient Synovitis Likely:

1. Afebrile, well-appearing, normal bloodwork
2. Supportive care: ibuprofen, acetaminophen
3. Rest and gradual return to activity
4. Close follow-up in 24–48 hours

Do Not:

1. Delay antibiotics in suspected septic arthritis
2. Attempt joint aspiration unless trained and safe to perform
3. Dismiss limp in a febrile child without workup

When to Refer

Immediate Transfer:

1. Suspected septic arthritis (high Kocher score)
2. Febrile child refusing to walk
3. Joint effusion on ultrasound with systemic signs
4. Positive blood cultures

Urgent Referral (1–3 days):

1. Unclear diagnosis with mild symptoms
2. Persistent limp despite treatment
3. No improvement in 48 hours

Routine Follow-up:

1. Classic transient synovitis with resolution
2. Normal bloodwork and afebrile child walking within 1– 2 days

Admission Orders

1. Admit to Rural Medicine – Suspected Septic Arthritis
2. Diagnosis: [e.g., suspected septic arthritis of hip]
3. Condition: Stable
4. Allergies: [Document here]

Orders:

1. Vitals q4h
2. NPO until seen by ortho
3. Bedrest and limb immobilization
4. IV Ceftriaxone 75 mg/kg/day divided q12h (max 2 g/day)
5. Acetaminophen 15 mg/kg PO q6h PRN
6. Morphine 0.1 mg/kg IV q4h PRN
7. Labs: CBC, ESR, CRP, blood cultures
8. Imaging: X-ray, joint ultrasound
9. Notify pediatric orthopedic surgeon
10. Discharge Plan: Transfer to tertiary center or improve and follow-up arranged

Rural ER Pearls

1. Septic joint is a true emergency; delay in treatment can lead to permanent joint damage.
2. Kocher criteria are helpful but not definitive; use clinical judgment.
3. Always do a thorough neurovascular and hip exam in any child with a limp.
4. Transient synovitis is self-limited, but requires follow-up to ensure resolution.
5. Consider alternative diagnoses (Perthes, fracture, malignancy) if symptoms persist.

SPINE & NECK

CHAPTER 25
Neck Injuries and Cervical Spine Precautions

Introduction

Cervical spine injuries can result in devastating neurologic outcomes. In rural emergency departments, prompt immobilization, careful assessment, and appropriate imaging are critical. This chapter focuses on common neck trauma presentations, red flags, spinal precautions, and safe disposition planning.

Assessment

History:

1. Mechanism: MVC, fall >3 ft, axial load, sports injury, assault
2. Neck pain, weakness, paresthesias
3. Loss of consciousness, distracting injuries
4. Use validated tools (e.g., Canadian C-Spine Rule)

Physical Exam:

1. Assess for midline tenderness
2. Range of motion only if cleared by decision rule
3. Neurologic exam: motor, sensory, reflexes
4. Check for signs of spinal cord injury: weakness, incontinence

Canadian C-Spine Rule (High-risk features):

1. Age ≥65
2. Dangerous mechanism (e.g., fall >3 ft, high-speed MVC)
3. Paresthesias in extremities

Low-risk features that allow safe ROM testing:

1. Ambulatory at any time
2. Delayed onset of neck pain
3. No midline tenderness
4. Sitting position in ED
5. Simple rear-end MVC

Imaging:

1. CT cervical spine (preferred for trauma)
2. X-ray if CT not available and low suspicion
3. MRI if neurologic deficits or suspected cord injury

Management

Spinal Precautions:

1. Apply rigid cervical collar immediately
2. Log roll for movement and transfer
3. Keep head midline and neutral
4. Maintain spinal precautions until cleared by imaging and assessment

Initial ED Management:

1. Ensure airway, breathing, circulation
2. Analgesia: acetaminophen, opioids PRN
3. Immobilize using board and collar
4. Assess for multisystem trauma
5. Consult regional trauma/neurosurgery early

Cervical Spine Clearance:

1. If imaging and neuro exam normal and low-risk criteria met: may remove collar
2. If imaging not available or abnormal: maintain collar and refer/transfer

Do Not:

1. Remove collar before full assessment and imaging
2. Use flexion/extension X-rays in the ED
3. Delay transfer for advanced imaging if neurologic signs present

When to Refer

Immediate Transfer:

1. Neurologic deficits
2. High suspicion of unstable cervical injury
3. Fracture on CT with or without symptoms
4. Inability to clear spine due to AMS or polytrauma

Urgent Referral (1–3 days):

1. Stable cervical fracture identified without neuro deficits
2. Persistent midline tenderness after normal X-ray

Routine Follow-up:

1. Strain or sprain injuries with normal imaging
2. Chronic neck pain without trauma or red flags

Admission Orders

1. Admit to Rural Medicine – Cervical Spine Injury
2. Diagnosis: Suspected C-spine fracture or high-risk mechanism
3. Condition: Stable
4. Allergies: [Document here]

Orders:

1. Vitals q4h, neuro checks q4h
2. Cervical collar to remain in place
3. Log roll precautions with all movements

4. Analgesia:
5. Acetaminophen 1000 mg PO q6h
6. Morphine 2–5 mg IV q4h PRN

Imaging:

1. CT cervical spine (if not already done)
2. MRI if neurologic deficits or spinal cord suspected
3. Labs: CBC, electrolytes if polytrauma
4. Referral: Neurosurgery or spine orthopedics
5. Discharge Plan: Spine cleared or stable, safe for transfer or follow-up arranged

Rural ER Pearls

1. Always assume cervical spine injury in trauma until proven otherwise.
2. Canadian C-Spine Rule is validated and reduces unnecessary imaging.
3. Use log roll and collar for all suspected injuries until cleared.
4. In obtunded or intoxicated patients, do not clear spine clinically—imaging is mandatory.
5. Early involvement of trauma/neuro services can expedite care and transfer.

CHAPTER 26
Red Flag Back Pain and Spinal Emergencies

Introduction

Back pain is a common complaint in the emergency department. While most cases are benign and self-limiting, certain presentations warrant urgent evaluation for serious underlying conditions. In rural emergency settings, recognizing red flags and initiating timely investigations or transfer is critical to prevent irreversible outcomes like paralysis or sepsis.

Assessment

History:

1. Mechanism: trauma, lifting, fall, spontaneous
2. Duration and progression of pain

Red Flag Symptoms:

1. Age >50 or <20
2. Night pain or weight loss
3. Fever, chills, recent infection
4. History of cancer
5. Trauma or recent surgery
6. IV drug use
7. Incontinence or saddle anesthesia

Physical Exam:

1. General appearance, fever
2. Inspection for deformity, bruising, tenderness
3. Palpation of spine
4. Motor strength in lower limbs
5. Reflexes: knee, ankle, Babinski
6. Sensory exam including perineum

7. Rectal tone and post-void residual if cauda equina suspected

Imaging:

1. X-ray for trauma, fracture, or malignancy
2. MRI (if available) for neurologic symptoms or suspected spinal cord compression
3. CT spine if MRI not available and fracture suspected
4. Labs: CBC, CRP/ESR, blood cultures (if infection suspected)

Management

Initial Management:

1. Analgesia: acetaminophen, NSAIDs, opioids, avoid excessive sedation
2. Consider IV dexamethasone 10 mg IV if spinal cord compression
3. Urgent bladder scan for retention
4. Foley catheter if cauda equina suspected and unable to void
5. IV antibiotics (e.g., ceftriaxone + vancomycin) if epidural abscess suspected

Do Not:

1. Delay transfer if red flags are present and MRI is not available
2. Miss subtle signs like new urinary hesitancy or gait instability

Common Emergencies:

1. Cauda equina syndrome: urinary retention, saddle anesthesia, bilateral leg weakness
2. Epidural abscess: fever + back pain + neurologic deficit

3. Spinal metastasis: progressive night pain, history of malignancy
4. Compression fractures: sudden pain in elderly or corticosteroid use

When to Refer

Immediate Transfer:

1. Suspected cauda equina syndrome
2. Epidural abscess
3. Progressive neurologic deficit
4. Spinal trauma with instability or fracture
5. Suspected spinal cord compression

Urgent Referral (1–3 days):

1. Vertebral osteomyelitis/discitis without instability
2. Malignancy with stable neurology
3. Significant compression fracture with persistent pain

Routine Follow-up:

1. Mechanical back pain without red flags
2. Chronic low back pain with preserved function
3. Follow-up with primary care or physio as needed

Admission Orders

1. Admit to Rural Medicine – Red Flag Back Pain
2. Diagnosis: Suspected cauda equina syndrome / Spinal metastasis / Compression fracture
3. Condition: Stable
4. Allergies: [Document here]

Orders:

1. Vitals q4h, neuro checks each shift
2. Analgesia:
3. Acetaminophen 1000 mg PO q6h
4. Morphine 2–5 mg IV q4h PRN
5. Foley catheter if urinary retention present
6. Dexamethasone 10 mg IV once, then 4 mg IV q6h if spinal cord compression
7. IV antibiotics if infection suspected:
8. Vancomycin + ceftriaxone
9. Labs: CBC, CRP, ESR, blood cultures
10. Imaging: MRI spine if available, otherwise CT and urgent transfer
11. Referral: Neurosurgery or orthopedic spine surgery
12. Discharge Plan: Transfer arranged or close outpatient follow-up with imaging pending

Rural ER Pearls

1. Back pain + urinary changes = assume cauda equina until ruled out.
2. Always ask about red flag symptoms and perform rectal exam when indicated.
3. MRI is the gold standard for cord compression, abscess, or malignancy.
4. Night pain and weight loss suggest malignancy or infection.
5. Don't overlook compression fractures in elderly with sudden pain after minor trauma.

SHOULDER & CLAVICLE
(INCL. PROXIMAL HUMERUS)

CHAPTER 27
Acromioclavicular (AC) Joint Injuries

Introduction

Acromioclavicular (AC) joint injuries are common shoulder injuries, typically resulting from direct trauma to the lateral shoulder, such as a fall onto the point of the shoulder or contact sports injury. They range from mild sprains to complete disruption of the AC and coracoclavicular (CC) ligaments. The Rockwood classification system (Types I–VI) helps guide management decisions. Early recognition and appropriate immobilization can prevent chronic instability and pain.

Assessment

History:

1. Mechanism: direct blow to the shoulder, fall onto point of shoulder, sports collision
2. Pain localized to AC joint
3. Difficulty lifting arm overhead
4. Previous shoulder injuries

Physical Exam:

1. Tenderness over AC joint
2. Swelling and localized deformity
3. Step-off at AC joint in higher-grade injuries
4. Pain with cross-body adduction test
5. Assess neurovascular status: radial pulse, sensation in upper limb

Imaging:

1. X-ray shoulder (AP and Zanca views)
2. Stress views (weights in hands) may help assess CC ligament disruption

Rockwood Classification:

1. Type I: Sprain of AC ligaments, no displacement
2. Type II: Rupture of AC ligaments, partial CC ligament injury, slight displacement
3. Type III: Complete rupture of AC and CC ligaments, significant displacement
4. Types IV–VI: Severe displacement, often requiring surgery

Management

Type I and II Injuries:

1. Sling immobilization for comfort (1–2 weeks)
2. Ice, rest, analgesia
3. Early physiotherapy to maintain range of motion

Type III Injuries:

1. Most can be treated non-operatively in rural setting with sling and physiotherapy
2. Consider orthopedic referral for high-demand athletes or persistent symptoms

Type IV–VI Injuries:

1. Require urgent orthopedic referral for surgical repair
2. Immobilization and pain control until transfer

General Principles:

1. Analgesia: acetaminophen, NSAIDs, opioids for severe pain
2. Avoid heavy lifting or overhead activities until cleared
3. Educate patient about gradual return to activity

When to Refer

Immediate Transfer:

1. Open injury over AC joint
2. Neurovascular compromise
3. Types IV–VI injuries

Urgent Referral (1–3 days):

1. Unstable Type III injuries in athletes or manual laborers
2. Persistent instability or pain despite conservative management

Routine Follow-up:

1. Type I and II injuries
2. Stable Type III injuries

Admission Orders

1. Admit to Rural Medicine – AC Joint Injury Observation
2. Diagnosis: Rockwood Type II AC joint separation
3. Condition: Stable
4. Allergies: [Document here]

Orders:

1. Vitals q4h
2. Analgesia:
3. Acetaminophen 1000 mg PO q6h
4. Ibuprofen 400 mg PO q6h

5. Morphine 2–5 mg SC q4h PRN
6. Immobilization: Sling for comfort
7. Ice application q2–3h while awake
8. Neurovascular checks q4h
9. Referral: Orthopedic surgery as indicated
10. Discharge Plan: Pain controlled, sling education, physiotherapy referral

Rural ER Pearls

1. Always compare both shoulders on imaging for subtle displacement
2. Rockwood classification helps guide management and referral urgency
3. Early physiotherapy is essential to prevent stiffness and chronic pain
4. Types IV–VI require surgery—arrange transfer if in rural setting

CHAPTER 28
Clavicle Fractures

Introduction

Clavicle fractures are common injuries, accounting for approximately 2.6–5% of all fractures and up to 44% of shoulder girdle fractures. They frequently occur in young adults following a fall onto the shoulder or direct trauma (e.g., sports injury, motor vehicle accident). In the rural emergency setting, rapid assessment, pain control, and safe disposition are key — especially given potential limitations in on-site orthopedic support.

Assessment

History:

1. Mechanism of injury (fall on outstretched arm, direct blow, MVC)
2. Dominant arm involved?
3. Neurologic symptoms: numbness, tingling, weakness?
4. Open wound or visible bone?
5. Associated injuries (rib fractures, scapula, head trauma)

Physical Exam:

1. Deformity, swelling, ecchymosis over the clavicle
2. Tenderness along the clavicle
3. Palpable "step-off" or mobility
4. Assess skin integrity — risk of open fracture or tenting

Neurovascular exam:

1. Check brachial plexus (motor/sensory)
2. Check axillary, radial, median, ulnar nerves
3. Radial pulse and capillary refill

107

Imaging:

1. X-ray clavicle (AP + 15° cephalic tilt) – standard
2. Consider chest X-ray if:
3. Suspected rib fracture or pneumothorax
4. Medial clavicle fracture (risk of great vessel injury)

Management

Conservative (Most Midshaft Fractures):

1. Immobilization with sling (or figure-of-eight if tolerated)
2. Analgesia: Acetaminophen, NSAIDs, consider short opioid course
3. Ice packs: 20 minutes every 2 hours during first 48 hours
4. Early mobilization: Pendulum exercises after 7–10 days; full ROM at 4–6 weeks
5. Return to activity: Full union in 6–12 weeks

Indications for Urgent Orthopedic Referral (Even if Rural):

1. Open fracture
2. Neurovascular compromise
3. Skin tenting (impending open fracture)
4. Severely displaced or comminuted midshaft fracture >2cm
5. Medial or lateral clavicle fractures (less common, higher complication rate)
6. Floating shoulder (clavicle + scapular neck fracture)
7. Non-union or delayed union on follow-up

When to Refer

Immediate Transfer (Stat):

1. Open fracture
2. Neurovascular injury

3. Skin tenting
4. Associated polytrauma (head, chest, spine)

Urgent Orthopedic Referral (1–3 days):

1. Highly displaced or shortened fractures
2. Bilateral clavicle fractures
3. Medial/lateral end fractures
4. Athletes or manual laborers needing faster return to function

Routine Outpatient Follow-up:

1. Non-displaced or minimally displaced midshaft fractures
2. No neurovascular compromise
3. Ensure follow-up with family physician or orthopedic service in 1–2 weeks

Admission Orders

1. Admit to Rural Medicine – Fracture Observation
2. Diagnosis: Closed displaced midshaft clavicle fracture
3. Condition: Stable
4. Allergies: [Document here]

Orders:

1. Vitals q4h
2. Analgesia:
3. Acetaminophen 1000 mg PO q6h PRN
4. Ibuprofen 400 mg PO q6h PRN
5. Morphine 2–5 mg SC q4h PRN severe pain
6. Immobilization: Apply arm sling or figure-of-eight bandage
7. Imaging: X-ray clavicle (repeat if concerns)
8. Neurovascular checks q4h x 24h

9. Activity: Bedrest with bathroom privileges; arm supported
10. Referral: Fax referral to orthopedic surgery, include images
11. Discharge Plan: Once pain controlled, clear discharge instructions, follow-up arranged

Rural ER Pearls

1. Most clavicle fractures heal non-operatively.
2. Skin tenting = treat like open fracture risk.
3. Medial clavicle fractures: rare, but risk of major vessel injury.
4. Document thorough neurovascular exam before and after immobilization.
5. Always provide clear discharge instructions for sling use and follow-up.

CHAPTER 29
Proximal Humerus Fractures

Introduction

Proximal humerus fractures are common in older adults, particularly postmenopausal women with osteoporosis. They often result from low-energy falls and may present subtly in the elderly. Prompt recognition, immobilization, and appropriate referral are critical in rural settings to minimize complications and restore function.

Assessment

History:

1. Mechanism: fall onto outstretched hand, direct blow to shoulder
2. Age and comorbidities (osteoporosis, dementia, anticoagulation)
3. Dominant arm involved?
4. Pain severity, functional limitation
5. Numbness, tingling, weakness suggesting nerve injury

Physical Exam:

1. Swelling, ecchymosis around the shoulder and upper arm
2. Arm held adducted against the body
3. Tenderness at proximal humerus
4. Limited range of motion, pain with passive movement
5. Assess axillary nerve: deltoid sensation and motor
6. Check radial pulse and capillary refill

Imaging:

1. X-ray shoulder (AP, scapular Y, axillary view)

2. CT scan if X-ray unclear and available (not routine in rural ER)
3. Consider additional imaging for elderly patients (e.g., hip, spine) if high fall mechanism

Management

Conservative Management (most non-displaced or minimally displaced fractures):

1. Immobilization with sling or shoulder immobilizer
2. Analgesia: Acetaminophen, NSAIDs; opioids short-term if severe pain
3. Ice and elevation
4. Initiate pendulum exercises after 7–10 days
5. Gradual return to function with physiotherapy

Surgical Referral Indications:

1. Displaced fractures >1 cm
2. 2-part, 3-part, or 4-part fractures (Neer classification)
3. Fracture-dislocation of the humeral head
4. Open fracture
5. Associated neurovascular injury
6. Failure of conservative treatment with ongoing dysfunction

When to Refer

Immediate Transfer:

1. Open fracture
2. Suspected humeral head fracture-dislocation
3. Neurovascular compromise

Urgent Orthopedic Referral (1–3 days):

1. Multi-part displaced fractures
2. Elderly patient with loss of function
3. Fractures involving the anatomical neck

Routine Follow-up:

1. Non-displaced fractures with intact neurovascular status
2. Follow-up in 7–10 days with family physician or orthopedic specialist

Admission Orders

1. Admit to Rural Medicine – Proximal Humerus Fracture
2. Diagnosis: Closed non-displaced proximal humerus fracture
3. Condition: Stable
4. Allergies: [Document here]

Orders:

1. Vitals q4h
2. Analgesia:
3. Acetaminophen 1000 mg PO q6h PRN
4. Ibuprofen 400 mg PO q6h PRN
5. Morphine 2–5 mg SC q4h PRN for severe pain
6. Immobilization: Apply shoulder immobilizer or sling
7. Imaging: Repeat X-ray if pain worsens or neurovascular change
8. Neurovascular checks q4h x 24h
9. Activity: Bedrest with assisted ambulation
10. Referral: Fax referral to orthopedic service if indicated
11. Discharge Plan: Pain controlled, follow-up instructions, sling education

Rural ER Pearls

1. Axillary nerve injury is the most common nerve injury with proximal humerus fractures—check deltoid sensation.
2. Most non-displaced fractures in the elderly can be managed conservatively.
3. Early mobilization and physiotherapy are key to preventing frozen shoulder.
4. Consider osteoporosis screening and fall prevention education in elderly patients.
5. Always reassess neurovascular status after immobilization.

CHAPTER 30
Rotator Cuff Tears (Acute Traumatic)

Introduction

Acute traumatic rotator cuff tears occur when one or more of the rotator cuff tendons (supraspinatus, infraspinatus, subscapularis, teres minor) are suddenly torn due to high-energy trauma or a fall onto an outstretched hand. These injuries are most common in middle-aged and older adults, often following shoulder dislocation or heavy lifting. Prompt recognition is essential because early surgical repair improves functional outcomes, especially in large or complete tears.

Assessment

History:

1. Mechanism: fall on outstretched hand, heavy lifting, shoulder dislocation
2. Sudden onset of shoulder pain
3. Weakness in lifting the arm or rotating the shoulder
4. Inability to perform overhead activities
5. History of prior shoulder problems

Physical Exam:

1. Limited active range of motion, particularly abduction and external rotation
2. Weakness on supraspinatus testing (empty can test)
3. Weakness on external rotation against resistance (infraspinatus)
4. Weakness on internal rotation (subscapularis, lift-off test)
5. Tenderness over greater tuberosity
6. Neurovascular exam: radial pulse, sensation over deltoid

Imaging:

1. X-ray shoulder: usually normal, may show associated fracture or dislocation
2. Ultrasound: useful in rural settings to detect tendon discontinuity
3. MRI: gold standard for diagnosis and preoperative planning

Management

General Approach:

1. Analgesia: acetaminophen, NSAIDs, opioids for severe pain
2. Sling for comfort (short-term)
3. Ice application and activity modification
4. Early physiotherapy for partial tears

Complete or Large Tears:

1. Require urgent orthopedic referral (within 1–2 weeks) for possible surgical repair
2. Keep shoulder immobilized until assessment

Partial Tears:

1. Conservative management with physiotherapy and gradual return to activity
2. Orthopedic follow-up recommended

When to Refer

Immediate Transfer:

1. Associated fracture-dislocation
2. Neurovascular compromise

Urgent Referral (within 1–2 weeks):

1. Complete tear confirmed on imaging
2. Large tear with significant functional loss

Routine Follow-up:

1. Small partial tear with preserved function

Admission Orders

1. Admit to Rural Medicine – Acute Rotator Cuff Tear
2. Diagnosis: Suspected complete rotator cuff tear
3. Condition: Stable
4. Allergies: [Document here]

Orders:

1. Vitals q4h
2. Analgesia:
3. Acetaminophen 1000 mg PO q6h
4. Ibuprofen 400 mg PO q6h
5. Morphine 2–5 mg SC q4h PRN
6. Immobilization: Sling for comfort
7. Ice application q2–3h
8. Imaging: Ultrasound or MRI as available
9. Neurovascular checks q4h
10. Referral: Orthopedic surgery as indicated
11. Discharge Plan: Pain controlled, sling education, follow-up arranged

Rural ER Pearls

1. High suspicion after shoulder trauma with weakness and preserved passive motion
2. Early surgical repair offers best outcomes for complete tears

3. Ultrasound is a useful rural diagnostic tool when MRI is unavailable
4. Do not delay referral in suspected complete tears

CHAPTER 31
Shoulder Dislocations

Introduction

Shoulder dislocations are among the most frequent large joint dislocations encountered in emergency medicine. The majority (over 95%) are anterior dislocations, often caused by a fall on an outstretched arm. In rural settings, prompt recognition, pain control, and timely reduction are essential to preserve joint function and minimize complications.

Assessment

History:

1. Mechanism of injury (fall, seizure, direct trauma)
2. First-time dislocation vs recurrent?
3. Arm position at the time of injury
4. Associated numbness, weakness, or paresthesia?
5. Prior reduction experience or complications?

Physical Exam:

1. Arm held in slight abduction and external rotation (anterior dislocation)
2. Prominent acromion, flattened shoulder contour
3. Palpable humeral head in subcoracoid or subglenoid position
4. Assess axillary nerve: deltoid sensation and function
5. Assess radial, ulnar, and median nerves; check distal pulses

Imaging:

1. X-ray shoulder (AP, lateral/Y-view, axillary view if tolerated)
2. Rule out associated fractures (greater tuberosity, Hill-Sachs, Bankart lesions)

Management

Pre-Reduction:

1. Informed consent and explanation
2. Neurovascular status documented pre- and post-reduction
3. IV access and monitoring if sedation is used
4. Analgesia: ketorolac, acetaminophen, or local intra-articular lidocaine
5. Procedural sedation if needed (midazolam/fentanyl or ketamine)

Reduction Techniques (select based on experience):

1. Stimson technique (gravity-assisted)
2. External rotation method
3. Traction-countertraction
4. Scapular manipulation (effective in elderly)

Post-Reduction:

1. Confirm reduction with repeat X-ray
2. Neurovascular reassessment
3. Sling or shoulder immobilizer
4. Early range of motion exercises after 1–2 weeks for older patients
5. Physiotherapy referral if available

When to Refer

Immediate Transfer:

1. Irreducible dislocation
2. Suspected fracture-dislocation
3. Neurovascular compromise that persists post-reduction

Urgent Orthopedic Follow-up (1–3 days):

1. Recurrent dislocations, especially in athletes
2. Greater tuberosity fracture
3. High-demand patients needing faster rehab

Routine Follow-up:

1. First-time uncomplicated dislocation with good reduction
2. Arrange follow-up in 7–10 days with primary care or orthopedics

Admission Orders

1. Admit to Rural Medicine – Shoulder Dislocation Observation
2. Diagnosis: Anterior shoulder dislocation (reduced)
3. Condition: Stable
4. Allergies: [Document here]

Orders:

1. Vitals q4h
2. Analgesia:
3. Acetaminophen 1000 mg PO q6h PRN
4. Ibuprofen 400 mg PO q6h PRN
5. Morphine 2–5 mg SC q4h PRN severe pain
6. Immobilization: Sling or shoulder immobilizer
7. Neurovascular checks q4h

8. Imaging: Post-reduction X-ray (if not done already)
9. Activity: Bedrest with bathroom privileges
10. Referral: Fax referral to orthopedic service if indicated
11. Discharge Plan: Discharge when pain controlled and safe transfer arranged

Rural ER Pearls

1. Always document neurovascular status before and after reduction.
2. Scapular manipulation is low-risk and effective without sedation.
3. First-time dislocators <30 years have a high recurrence rate.
4. Intra-articular lidocaine is a safe alternative to sedation in resource-limited settings.
5. Consider early mobilization in elderly patients to avoid frozen shoulder.

ELBOW & FOREARM

CHAPTER 32
Elbow Injuries

Introduction

Elbow injuries, including dislocations and supracondylar fractures, are common in both adults and children. Posterior elbow dislocations are typically due to falls on an outstretched arm, while supracondylar fractures are more common in children aged 5–7 years. Prompt assessment and reduction are critical to prevent long-term complications such as neurovascular injury or compartment syndrome.

Assessment

History:

1. Mechanism of injury (fall, direct blow, twisting injury)
2. Age of patient (supracondylar fractures more common in young children)
3. Pain location and inability to move elbow
4. Neurologic symptoms: numbness, tingling
5. Hand function and circulation

Physical Exam:

1. Obvious deformity, swelling, ecchymosis around elbow
2. Limited or no range of motion
3. Assess distal pulses (brachial, radial, ulnar)
4. Check median, radial, and ulnar nerve function
5. Look for signs of compartment syndrome (pain out of proportion, firm compartments)

Imaging:

1. X-ray elbow (AP and lateral)
2. Fat pad sign may indicate occult fracture

3. In children, look for anterior humeral line and radiocapitellar alignment

Management

Elbow Dislocation (usually posterior):

1. Pre-reduction neurovascular exam
2. Procedural sedation or intra-articular anesthesia
3. Reduction technique: traction and counter-traction with gradual elbow flexion
4. Post-reduction X-ray to confirm alignment
5. Sling immobilization for 1–2 weeks
6. Early range of motion to prevent stiffness

Supracondylar Fractures (especially in children):

1. Type I (non-displaced): immobilization with posterior splint
2. Type II–III (displaced): require orthopedic consultation and likely surgical fixation
3. Monitor for signs of compartment syndrome
4. Avoid circumferential casting in acute swelling

Analgesia:

1. Acetaminophen, NSAIDs, opioids for severe pain
2. Elevation and ice

When to Refer

Immediate Transfer:

1. Absent pulses or vascular compromise
2. Open fracture
3. Compartment syndrome
4. Displaced supracondylar fracture
5. Irreducible dislocation

Urgent Orthopedic Referral (1–3 days):

1. Dislocated joint with good neurovascular function after reduction
2. Minimally displaced supracondylar fracture in children

Routine Follow-up:

1. Type I supracondylar fracture or reduced elbow dislocation
2. Stable neurovascular status
3. Follow-up in 7–10 days

Admission Orders

1. Admit to Rural Medicine – Elbow Injury Observation
2. Diagnosis: Posterior elbow dislocation / Supracondylar fracture
3. Condition: Stable
4. Allergies: [Document here]

Orders:

1. Vitals q4h
2. Analgesia:
3. Acetaminophen 1000 mg PO q6h PRN
4. Ibuprofen 400 mg PO q6h PRN
5. Morphine 2–5 mg SC q4h PRN
6. Immobilization: Posterior splint in 90° flexion if tolerated
7. Imaging: Repeat X-ray post-reduction or if worsening pain
8. Neurovascular checks q4h
9. Elevate limb and apply ice packs
10. Referral: Fax orthopedic referral if indicated
11. Discharge Plan: Once pain is controlled and follow-up arranged

Rural ER Pearls

1. Always document neurovascular status before and after any reduction.
2. In children, assess anterior humeral line and fat pad signs carefully on X-ray.
3. Early mobilization prevents elbow stiffness in dislocation cases.
4. Type III supracondylar fractures are surgical emergencies due to high risk of neurovascular compromise.
5. Beware of evolving compartment syndrome in high-energy elbow trauma

CHAPTER 33
Forearm Fractures

Introduction

Forearm fractures are common injuries and may involve the radius, ulna, or both bones. These injuries often result from falls, direct trauma, or twisting mechanisms. Monteggia and Galeazzi fractures are named fracture-dislocation patterns that require special attention. In rural emergency settings, identifying the pattern and stabilizing the limb for timely referral is essential to prevent complications such as compartment syndrome, malunion, or chronic instability.

Assessment

History:

1. Mechanism of injury: fall, motor vehicle collision, sports injury
2. Location of pain, deformity, and functional loss
3. Neurologic symptoms: numbness, weakness, paresthesia
4. Dominant hand involved?
5. Pediatric vs adult forearm fracture context

Physical Exam:

1. Visible deformity, swelling, tenderness along radius and ulna
2. Palpable crepitus or step-off
3. Assess wrist and elbow joints for associated dislocation
4. Neurovascular exam:
5. Radial, median, ulnar nerve function
6. Capillary refill and distal pulses

Imaging:

1. X-ray forearm (AP and lateral views) including both elbow and wrist
2. Monteggia: Proximal ulna fracture + radial head dislocation
3. Galeazzi: Distal radius fracture + distal radioulnar joint (DRUJ) dislocation
4. Ensure joint alignment proximally and distally

Management

General Principles:

1. Immobilize the limb with a well-padded long arm posterior splint
2. Elevation and ice
3. Pain control with NSAIDs, acetaminophen, or opioids
4. Tetanus update and antibiotics if open fracture
5. Conservative (rarely used unless pediatric, non-displaced, or stable fracture):
6. Immobilization alone may suffice in some pediatric greenstick or buckle fractures

Surgical Referral Indications:

1. All displaced or angulated fractures in adults
2. Open fractures
3. Monteggia and Galeazzi fractures
4. Neurovascular compromise
5. Unstable reduction or failure to maintain alignment

When to Refer

Immediate Transfer:

1. Open fracture
2. Neurovascular compromise
3. Monteggia or Galeazzi fracture-dislocations
4. Suspected compartment syndrome

Urgent Orthopedic Referral (1–3 days):

1. Displaced both-bone fractures
2. Unstable single bone fracture with wrist/elbow involvement

Routine Follow-up:

1. Non-displaced or pediatric buckle fractures
2. Ensure X-ray reassessment and follow-up in 7–10 days

Admission Orders

1. Admit to Rural Medicine – Forearm Fracture Observation
2. Diagnosis: Both-bone forearm fracture / Monteggia / Galeazzi fracture
3. Condition: Stable
4. Allergies: [Document here]

Orders:

1. Vitals q4h
2. Analgesia:
3. Acetaminophen 1000 mg PO q6h PRN
4. Ibuprofen 400 mg PO q6h PRN
5. Morphine 2–5 mg SC q4h PRN for severe pain
6. Immobilization: Long arm posterior splint, wrist in neutral, elbow at 90°

RURAL ORTHOPEDIC EMERGENCY POCKET GUIDE

7. Imaging: Repeat X-ray if worsening pain or neurovascular changes
8. Neurovascular checks q4h
9. Activity: Bedrest with limb elevation
10. Referral: Orthopedic referral with imaging attached
11. Discharge Plan: Stable for transfer or outpatient follow-up

Rural ER Pearls

1. Always obtain X-rays of both wrist and elbow in forearm trauma to avoid missing Monteggia or Galeazzi injuries.
2. Monteggia = ulna fracture + radial head dislocation; Galeazzi = radius fracture + DRUJ dislocation.
3. Early reduction and immobilization reduce the risk of compartment syndrome and malalignment.
4. Pediatric fractures often require less aggressive intervention than adults.
5. Missed Monteggia injuries can result in long-term dysfunction—always assess radial head alignment in children.

WRIST & HAND

CHAPTER 34
Scaphoid Fractures

Introduction

Scaphoid fractures are the most common carpal bone fractures, typically occurring after a fall on an outstretched hand (FOOSH). They are clinically important due to their risk of nonunion and avascular necrosis, particularly in proximal pole fractures. These injuries may be subtle on initial X-rays, so a high index of suspicion and proper immobilization are crucial in rural emergency settings.

Assessment

History:

1. Mechanism: Fall on an outstretched hand, sports injury, motor vehicle collision
2. Pain in radial side of wrist
3. Decreased grip strength
4. History of previous wrist injuries

Physical Exam:

1. Tenderness in the anatomic snuffbox
2. Tenderness on axial compression of thumb
3. Pain with wrist extension and radial deviation
4. Assess for swelling or bruising over the dorsoradial wrist
5. Neurovascular exam: radial pulse, capillary refill, median nerve sensation

Imaging:

1. X-ray wrist (PA, lateral, and scaphoid views)
2. If initial films are negative but suspicion is high → immobilize and arrange repeat imaging in 10–14 days
3. Consider CT or MRI if available for high suspicion and negative X-ray
4. Fracture classification: distal pole, waist, proximal pole (proximal fractures have higher risk of nonunion)

Management

General Approach:

1. RICE: rest, ice, compression, elevation
2. Immobilization with a thumb spica splint or cast
3. Analgesia: acetaminophen, NSAIDs, opioids if severe pain
4. Educate patient on avoiding wrist strain

Non-Displaced Fractures:

1. Distal pole or waist fractures: usually managed with immobilization and orthopedic follow-up
2. Immobilize in thumb spica for 6–12 weeks

Displaced or Proximal Pole Fractures:

1. Higher risk of nonunion or AVN
2. Early orthopedic referral; surgical fixation often required

Do Not:

1. Miss subtle fractures—always immobilize if in doubt
2. Rely solely on initial X-ray if symptoms and mechanism are suspicious

When to Refer

Immediate Transfer:

1. Open fracture
2. Associated perilunate dislocation or carpal instability
3. Neurovascular compromise

Urgent Referral (1–3 days):

1. Displaced fractures (>1 mm displacement)
2. Proximal pole fractures
3. Nonunion on follow-up imaging

Routine Follow-up:

1. Non-displaced waist or distal fractures with immobilization
2. Follow-up in 1–2 weeks with repeat imaging

Admission Orders

1. Admit to Rural Medicine – Scaphoid Fracture Observation
2. Diagnosis: Non-displaced waist scaphoid fracture
3. Condition: Stable
4. Allergies: [Document here]

Orders:

1. Vitals q4h
2. Analgesia:
3. Acetaminophen 1000 mg PO q6h
4. Ibuprofen 400 mg PO q6h
5. Morphine 2–5 mg SC q4h PRN
6. Immobilization: Thumb spica splint or cast
7. Elevate limb, ice pack application
8. Imaging: Repeat X-ray or CT if unclear diagnosis

9. Neurovascular checks q4h
10. Referral: Orthopedic surgery as indicated
11. Discharge Plan: Pain controlled, splint education, follow-up arranged

Rural ER Pearls

1. Always check for snuffbox tenderness after wrist trauma
2. Negative X-ray does not rule out fracture—immobilize if suspicious
3. Proximal fractures have the highest risk of AVN and require early referral
4. Thumb spica splint is the immobilization of choice
5. Educate patients about prolonged healing times and importance of follow-up

CHAPTER 35
Wrist Fractures

Introduction

Wrist fractures are among the most common fractures seen in the emergency department, particularly following falls onto an outstretched hand. Colles' and Smith's fractures involve the distal radius, while scaphoid fractures carry a high risk of non-union and avascular necrosis if missed. Prompt identification and immobilization are critical in rural settings to ensure appropriate outcomes.

Assessment

History:

1. Mechanism: Fall on outstretched hand (FOOSH), direct impact
2. Hand dominance
3. Immediate swelling or deformity
4. Ability to move wrist or fingers
5. Numbness or tingling (median nerve involvement)

Physical Exam:

1. Deformity and swelling at distal forearm or snuffbox tenderness
2. Check capillary refill and distal pulses
3. Palpate anatomical snuffbox (for scaphoid)
4. Sensory and motor exam of median, radial, and ulnar nerves

Imaging:

1. X-ray wrist (PA, lateral, oblique)
2. Colles': dorsal displacement of distal radius
3. Smith's: volar displacement of distal radius
4. Scaphoid fracture: may not be visible early; consider repeat X-ray or MRI in 10–14 days

Management

Colles' and Smith's Fractures:

1. Closed reduction if displaced (traction and manipulation)
2. Immobilization with sugar-tong or volar forearm splint
3. Elevation and ice
4. Analgesia: NSAIDs, acetaminophen, opioids if severe
5. Post-reduction X-ray to confirm alignment

Scaphoid Fracture:

1. Suspected fracture with snuffbox tenderness → treat as fracture
2. Immobilize with thumb spica splint even if initial X-ray is normal
3. Arrange follow-up imaging or orthopedic consult in 10–14 days

Surgical Referral Indications:

1. Open fracture
2. Intra-articular displacement
3. Comminuted or unstable distal radius fractures
4. Scaphoid fractures with displacement
5. Neurovascular compromise

When to Refer

Immediate Transfer:

1. Open fracture
2. Neurovascular compromise
3. Irreducible fracture-dislocation

Urgent Orthopedic Referral (1–3 days):

1. Displaced distal radius fracture
2. Suspected scaphoid fracture requiring MRI/CT
3. Unstable fracture pattern

Routine Follow-up:

1. Non-displaced distal radius fracture in good alignment
2. Snuffbox tenderness with normal X-ray (scaphoid)
3. Follow-up in 7–10 days with repeat imaging if needed

Admission Orders

1. Admit to Rural Medicine – Wrist Fracture
2. Diagnosis: Displaced distal radius fracture / Suspected scaphoid fracture
3. Condition: Stable
4. Allergies: [Document here]

Orders:

1. Vitals q4h
2. Analgesia:
3. Acetaminophen 1000 mg PO q6h PRN
4. Ibuprofen 400 mg PO q6h PRN
5. Morphine 2–5 mg SC q4h PRN
6. Immobilization: Sugar-tong splint (radius fracture) or thumb spica (scaphoid)
7. Imaging: Repeat X-ray post-reduction if applicable

8. Neurovascular checks q4h
9. Activity: Bedrest with limb elevated
10. Referral: Orthopedic consultation or follow-up referral
11. Discharge Plan: Pain controlled, splint education, follow-up arranged

Rural ER Pearls

1. Always suspect a scaphoid fracture with snuffbox tenderness—even with normal X-ray.
2. Colles' fracture is most common in elderly patients from low-energy falls.
3. Volar (Smith's) fractures are less common but may indicate high-energy trauma.
4. Reduction should be followed by confirmation imaging.
5. Median nerve compression may occur with distal radius fractures—monitor for paresthesia or weakness.

CHAPTER 36
Hand Fractures

Introduction

Hand fractures are common injuries seen in both emergency and primary care settings. These include metacarpal fractures (especially the fifth metacarpal or "Boxer's fracture") and phalangeal fractures. Most are caused by direct trauma such as punches, crush injuries, or falls. In rural settings, prompt diagnosis, proper splinting, and early identification of referral needs are essential to preserve hand function.

Assessment

History:

1. Mechanism: punch, crush, fall, work-related trauma
2. Dominant hand involved?
3. Pain, swelling, deformity, or inability to move fingers
4. History of similar injury or arthritis?
5. Tetanus status if open wound present

Physical Exam:

1. Swelling, deformity, or bruising over hand or fingers
2. Rotation of fingers (check with fist closure)
3. Open wounds or exposed bone
4. Neurovascular exam:
5. Capillary refill
6. Sensation (median, ulnar, radial nerves)
7. Motor testing (flexion, extension, abduction)

Imaging:

1. X-ray hand (PA, oblique, lateral views)
2. Boxer's fracture: transverse fracture of 5th metacarpal neck with volar angulation
3. Look for intra-articular extension or comminution

Management

Conservative:

1. Most metacarpal neck fractures (e.g., Boxer's) can be treated with ulnar gutter splint
2. Acceptable angulation:
3. 5th metacarpal: up to 40–50°
4. 4th: 30°
5. 2nd/3rd: <10°
6. Buddy taping for stable, non-displaced phalangeal fractures
7. Ice, elevation, and analgesia
8. Tetanus update and antibiotics for open fractures

Surgical Referral Indications:

1. Rotational deformity
2. Open fracture
3. Intra-articular involvement
4. Significant displacement or angulation exceeding accepted limits
5. Multiple fractures or associated tendon injuries

When to Refer

Immediate Transfer:

1. Open fracture with exposed bone
2. Irreducible dislocation or fracture

3. Neurovascular compromise
4. Crush injury with suspected compartment syndrome

Urgent Orthopedic Referral (1–3 days):

1. Rotational deformity
2. Intra-articular or comminuted fractures
3. Unstable fracture after splinting

Routine Follow-up:

1. Simple Boxer's fracture or non-displaced phalangeal fracture
2. Follow-up in 7–10 days with repeat imaging and functional assessment

Admission Orders

1. Admit to Rural Medicine – Hand Fracture Observation
2. Diagnosis: Closed Boxer's fracture / Phalangeal fracture
3. Condition: Stable
4. Allergies: [Document here]

Orders:

1. Vitals q4h
2. Analgesia:
3. Acetaminophen 1000 mg PO q6h PRN
4. Ibuprofen 400 mg PO q6h PRN
5. Morphine 2–5 mg SC q4h PRN if severe
6. Immobilization: Ulnar gutter splint (for 4th/5th metacarpal), buddy taping if appropriate
7. Imaging: Repeat hand X-ray if needed
8. Neurovascular checks q4h
9. Activity: Hand elevation, no weight-bearing
10. Referral: Fax to orthopedic or hand specialist if indicated

11. Discharge Plan: Pain controlled, splint education, outpatient follow-up arranged

Rural ER Pearls

1. Always assess for rotational deformity—ask patient to make a fist and look for finger overlap.
2. Acceptable angulation varies by metacarpal—don't over-reduce 5th metacarpal neck fractures unnecessarily.
3. Splinting technique matters—use padded ulnar gutter splint to protect function and prevent stiffness.
4. Watch for infection in open hand injuries, especially human bites (clenched fist injuries).
5. Missed rotational deformity leads to significant hand dysfunction long-term.

HIP & PELVIS

CHAPTER 37
Hip Dislocations

Introduction

Hip dislocations are orthopedic emergencies typically caused by high-energy trauma, such as motor vehicle collisions. The majority are posterior dislocations, which carry a risk of sciatic nerve injury and avascular necrosis if not promptly reduced. In rural emergency settings, urgent diagnosis, stabilization, and reduction (if safe and trained) are key to preserving joint function and minimizing complications.

Assessment

History:

1. Mechanism: dashboard injury (posterior), fall from height, MVC
2. Time since injury
3. Previous hip surgery or dislocation?
4. Pain severity and inability to bear weight

Physical Exam:

1. Posterior dislocation: leg is shortened, internally rotated, and adducted
2. Anterior dislocation: leg is externally rotated and abducted
3. Palpable femoral head (anterior dislocation)
4. Assess neurovascular status:
5. Sciatic nerve (dorsiflexion, plantarflexion, foot sensation)
6. Distal pulses and capillary refill

Imaging:

1. X-ray pelvis and affected hip (AP and lateral views)
2. Assess for associated fractures (femoral head, acetabulum, neck)
3. CT scan post-reduction to assess for intra-articular fragments (if available)

Management

Initial Management:

1. Assess and document neurovascular status
2. Administer analgesia and sedation if performing reduction
3. Reduce within 6 hours to minimize avascular necrosis risk
4. Closed reduction techniques:
5. Allis, Bigelow, or Stimson techniques
6. Ensure sufficient muscle relaxation and assistance

Post-Reduction:

1. Confirm reduction with repeat X-ray
2. Reassess neurovascular status
3. Immobilize with knee immobilizer or traction
4. Monitor for recurrent dislocation or nerve deficit

Avoid Reduction If:

1. Suspected associated fracture
2. Lack of adequate sedation or support
3. Transfer to tertiary care is imminent and safe

When to Refer

Immediate Transfer:

1. Associated fracture-dislocation (acetabular or femoral head)
2. Irreducible dislocation
3. Neurovascular compromise
4. Open dislocation
5. Lack of resources to safely sedate/reduce

Urgent Referral (1–2 days):

1. Reduced dislocation with stable vitals and normal neurovascular exam
2. Arrange follow-up imaging and orthopedic consultation

Routine Follow-up:

1. Not applicable — all cases require orthopedic assessment post-reduction

Admission Orders

1. Admit to Rural Medicine – Hip Dislocation (Reduced)
2. Diagnosis: Posterior hip dislocation (reduced)
3. Condition: Stable
4. Allergies: [Document here]

Orders:

1. Vitals q4h
2. IV access and fluids PRN
3. Analgesia:
4. Acetaminophen 1000 mg PO q6h
5. Morphine 2–5 mg IV q4h PRN
6. Imaging: Pre- and post-reduction X-rays
7. Neurovascular checks q2h x 12h, then q4h

8. Immobilization: Knee immobilizer on affected side
9. Activity: Bedrest until transfer or follow-up plan
10. Referral: Orthopedic surgery for evaluation and possible CT
11. Discharge Plan: Follow-up confirmed, pain managed, no neurovascular concerns

Rural ER Pearls

1. Time is critical — aim to reduce within 6 hours of injury to prevent avascular necrosis.
2. Posterior dislocations are more common and often occur from dashboard injuries.
3. Always check for associated acetabular or femoral fractures before attempting reduction.
4. Post-reduction neurovascular exam is mandatory.
5. Use appropriate sedation and multiple assistants for safe closed reduction.

CHAPTER 38
Hip Fractures

Introduction

Hip fractures are common in the elderly population and often result from low-energy falls. They are associated with significant morbidity, mortality, and functional decline. The two main types are intracapsular (femoral neck) and extracapsular (intertrochanteric). In rural emergency settings, early recognition, pain management, and transfer for surgical repair are essential for optimal outcomes.

Assessment

History:

1. Mechanism: fall from standing, twisting injury, direct blow
2. Sudden inability to bear weight
3. Comorbidities: osteoporosis, dementia, anticoagulation
4. Medications: anticoagulants, sedatives

Physical Exam:

1. Affected leg shortened and externally rotated
2. Pain with any movement of the hip or leg
3. Check for bruising over lateral hip or groin
4. Palpate femoral pulses
5. Neurological exam of lower limb (sensation, movement)

Imaging:

1. X-ray pelvis and affected hip (AP and lateral views)
2. Consider femur and spine X-rays if high suspicion with negative hip films

3. CT scan if X-rays are inconclusive but high clinical suspicion

Management

Initial Management:

1. Pain control: acetaminophen, NSAIDs, opioids, femoral nerve block if trained
2. Immobilization and gentle handling to avoid further displacement
3. IV fluids to maintain hydration
4. Monitor for delirium and hypotension in elderly

Surgical Referral:

1. All hip fractures require orthopedic surgical evaluation
2. Intracapsular fractures (femoral neck): often need hemiarthroplasty or total hip replacement
3. Intertrochanteric fractures: managed with ORIF (open reduction internal fixation)

Anticoagulation:

1. Assess bleeding risk and reverse anticoagulation if needed pre-op
2. Coordinate with surgical team regarding timing of surgery

When to Refer

Immediate Transfer:

1. All confirmed or suspected hip fractures
2. Inability to bear weight with deformity and pain
3. Suspected femoral neck fracture in elderly

Urgent Referral (within 24 hours):

1. Stable patients awaiting transport
2. Patients with pain but no radiographic fracture but high clinical suspicion

Routine Follow-up:

1. Not applicable — all patients require surgical evaluation

Admission Orders

1. Admit to Rural Medicine – Hip Fracture
2. Diagnosis: Suspected intertrochanteric hip fracture
3. Condition: Stable
4. Allergies: [Document here]

Orders:

1. Vitals q4h, monitor for delirium or hypotension
2. IV fluids: Normal saline at 75 mL/hr
3. Analgesia:
4. Acetaminophen 1000 mg PO q6h
5. Morphine 2–5 mg SC q4h PRN
6. NPO for potential surgery
7. Imaging: AP/lateral hip X-ray and pelvis
8. Labs: CBC, electrolytes, INR/PTT, group and screen
9. Foley catheter if urinary retention or immobility
10. Referral: Orthopedic surgery at nearest center
11. Discharge Plan: Transfer when medically optimized and transport arranged

Rural ER Pearls

1. Elderly patients with inability to bear weight after a fall should be treated as a hip fracture until proven otherwise.
2. Intracapsular fractures risk avascular necrosis and require prompt surgical input.
3. Consider occult hip fracture in patients with groin pain and negative X-ray—CT or MRI may be needed.
4. Early pain control reduces delirium risk in elderly patients.
5. Document pre-injury mobility and cognitive status for surgical planning.

CHAPTER 39
Pelvic Fractures

Introduction

Pelvic fractures are potentially life-threatening injuries often associated with high-energy trauma, such as motor vehicle collisions or falls from height. They can result in massive hemorrhage, bladder or urethral injury, and require urgent stabilization. In rural emergency settings, rapid identification, resuscitation, and timely transfer are crucial to improve outcomes.

Assessment

History:

1. Mechanism: high-speed trauma, fall from height, crush injury
2. Associated symptoms: hematuria, abdominal pain, leg weakness
3. Past pelvic surgeries or orthopedic history

Physical Exam:

1. Hemodynamic instability (hypotension, tachycardia)
2. Pelvic instability on compression (gentle anteroposterior and lateral pressure)
3. Ecchymosis over perineum, sacrum, or scrotum/labia
4. Leg length discrepancy or rotated lower limb
5. Neurological exam for lower limb deficits
6. Genitourinary exam: blood at urethral meatus, perineal hematoma, high-riding prostate

Imaging:

1. Portable AP pelvis X-ray (initial trauma screen)
2. CT abdomen/pelvis with contrast (if stable)
3. FAST exam to assess for intraperitoneal bleeding
4. Retrograde urethrogram if urethral injury suspected

Management

Initial Resuscitation:

1. Activate trauma protocol
2. 2 large bore IVs, isotonic fluid bolus
3. Type and crossmatch for transfusion
4. Apply pelvic binder over greater trochanters to reduce hemorrhage
5. Avoid repeated pelvic exams after binder placement

Adjunctive Measures:

1. Foley catheter unless urethral injury suspected
2. Monitor urine output and hematuria
3. IV analgesia and antiemetics
4. Monitor for signs of shock, abdominal compartment syndrome

Surgical Referral Indications:

1. All unstable pelvic fractures
2. Ongoing bleeding despite resuscitation
3. Associated abdominal or genitourinary injury

Do Not:

1. Delay transfer for definitive imaging or procedures in unstable patients

When to Refer

Immediate Transfer:

1. Hemodynamic instability with pelvic fracture
2. Suspected open pelvic fracture
3. Urologic injury (blood at meatus, high-riding prostate)
4. Complex or comminuted fractures requiring orthopedic trauma care

Urgent Referral (1–2 days if stable):

1. Minimally displaced stable fractures
2. Isolated pubic rami fracture with normal vitals (consider outpatient follow-up)

Routine Follow-up:

1. Non-displaced low-impact pelvic fractures in elderly with stable vitals
2. Consider outpatient PT, fall risk assessment

Admission Orders

1. Admit to Rural Medicine – Pelvic Fracture
2. Diagnosis: Pelvic ring fracture, hemodynamically stable
3. Condition: Stable
4. Allergies: [Document here]

Orders:

1. Vitals q1h, monitor for hypotension or tachycardia
2. IV fluids: Normal saline 1L bolus, then maintenance
3. Type and crossmatch 2 units PRBC
4. Analgesia:
5. Acetaminophen 1000 mg PO q6h
6. Morphine 2–5 mg IV q4h PRN
7. Apply pelvic binder if not already in place

8. NPO status if transfer planned
9. Foley catheter (unless urethral injury suspected)
10. Imaging: AP pelvis X-ray, FAST, CT if stable
11. Referral: Ortho-trauma and/or urology
12. Discharge Plan: Transfer when stabilized or follow-up arranged if non-transferable

Rural ER Pearls

1. Apply pelvic binder early over greater trochanters to reduce bleeding.
2. Don't delay transfer for full CT if patient is unstable—start resuscitation first.
3. Always consider genitourinary injuries in pelvic trauma—look for blood at the urethral meatus.
4. Avoid repeated manipulation of pelvis once a binder is applied.
5. Falls in elderly with pubic rami fractures can often be managed conservatively with pain control and mobilization.

FEMUR & THIGH

CHAPTER 40
Femoral Shaft Fractures

Introduction

Femoral shaft fractures are high-energy injuries typically resulting from motor vehicle collisions or falls from height. They can lead to significant blood loss, pain, and complications such as fat embolism or compartment syndrome. In rural emergency settings, early stabilization, pain control, and timely transfer for surgical fixation are critical.

Assessment

History:

1. Mechanism: high-energy trauma (MVC, fall from height)
2. Time since injury and associated symptoms
3. Past orthopedic history, use of bisphosphonates or osteoporosis

Physical Exam:

1. Obvious thigh deformity, swelling, and bruising
2. Shortened and externally rotated limb
3. Assess for open wounds or bleeding
4. Neurovascular exam: femoral pulse, distal pulses, motor/sensory function
5. Assess for associated injuries: pelvis, hip, knee, head, chest

Imaging:

1. X-ray femur (AP and lateral views)
2. Consider imaging of hip, knee, pelvis for associated fractures
3. CT trauma series if polytrauma suspected (if available)

159

Management

Initial Management:

1. ABCs and trauma protocol if multiple injuries
2. Pain control: IV opioids, acetaminophen, NSAIDs
3. Apply traction splint (e.g., Hare, Sager) if trained
4. Immobilize limb and elevate
5. IV fluids to support volume status
6. Monitor for signs of fat embolism: hypoxia, confusion, petechiae

Open Fractures:

1. Cover with sterile moist dressing
2. Initiate IV antibiotics and tetanus prophylaxis
3. Do not attempt definitive wound closure

Surgical Referral:

1. All femoral shaft fractures require surgical fixation (usually IM nailing)

When to Refer

Immediate Transfer:

1. Open femur fracture
2. Hemodynamic instability or signs of shock
3. Suspected fat embolism
4. Polytrauma requiring trauma team evaluation

Urgent Referral (within 24 hours):

1. Closed femur fracture in stable patient
2. Pain managed and traction applied

Routine Follow-up:

1. Not applicable — all cases require orthopedic surgery

Admission Orders

1. Admit to Rural Medicine – Femoral Shaft Fracture
2. Diagnosis: Closed midshaft femoral fracture
3. Condition: Stable
4. Allergies: [Document here]

Orders:

1. Vitals q2h, monitor for signs of bleeding or fat embolism
2. IV fluids: Normal saline 1L bolus, then 100 mL/hr
3. Analgesia:
4. Acetaminophen 1000 mg PO q6h
5. Morphine 5 mg IV q4h PRN
6. Apply traction splint if trained and available
7. Imaging: AP/lateral femur, hip, pelvis, knee X-rays
8. Labs: CBC, electrolytes, INR/PTT, crossmatch
9. Antibiotics: Cefazolin 2 g IV q8h if open fracture
10. Tetanus prophylaxis PRN
11. Referral: Orthopedic surgery for fixation
12. Discharge Plan: Stable vitals, pain controlled, transfer arranged

Rural ER Pearls

1. Femur fractures can cause up to 1.5 L of blood loss into the thigh — monitor closely.
2. Apply traction splint early to reduce bleeding and pain.
3. Always check for concurrent hip, knee, or pelvic injuries.
4. Watch for fat embolism syndrome within 24–72 hours of injury.

5. Document distal pulses and neurovascular status before and after splinting.

KNEE & PATELLA

CHAPTER 41
Knee Injuries

Introduction

Knee injuries are common presentations to rural emergency departments, particularly from sports injuries, falls, and motor vehicle accidents. They may involve ligament sprains or tears, patellar dislocation, meniscal injuries, and tibial plateau fractures. Timely identification and stabilization are crucial to preserve joint function and avoid long-term disability.

Assessment

History:

1. Mechanism: twisting, hyperextension, direct blow, fall
2. Ability to bear weight
3. Sensation of popping, locking, or instability
4. Previous knee injuries or surgeries

Physical Exam:

1. Inspection for swelling, deformity, effusion
2. Palpation for tenderness (joint line, tibial plateau, patella)
3. Assess for patellar tracking and position
4. Perform Lachman, anterior/posterior drawer, varus/valgus stress (if not too painful)
5. Assess range of motion if tolerable
6. Neurovascular exam: dorsalis pedis, posterior tibial pulses, peroneal nerve (foot dorsiflexion)

Imaging:

1. X-ray knee (AP, lateral, sunrise)
2. Ottawa Knee Rules for imaging:
3. Age ≥55
4. Tenderness at head of fibula or patella
5. Inability to flex to 90°
6. Inability to bear weight for 4 steps
7. CT for suspected tibial plateau fracture (if available)

Management

Ligamentous Injuries:

1. RICE: rest, ice, compression, elevation
2. Immobilization in knee brace or posterior splint
3. Crutches if unable to bear weight
4. NSAIDs or acetaminophen for pain
5. Outpatient MRI referral if ongoing instability

Patellar Dislocation:

1. Often lateral dislocation
2. Reduce with gentle extension of knee and medial pressure on patella
3. Post-reduction X-ray to rule out fracture or loose body
4. Immobilize with knee immobilizer for 2–3 weeks
5. Follow-up with physiotherapy

Tibial Plateau Fracture:

1. Non-weight-bearing, long leg splint
2. Analgesia, elevation
3. Urgent orthopedic referral for operative consideration

Avoid:

1. Stress testing acutely if major swelling or fracture suspected
2. Aggressive manipulation without imaging if dislocation or fracture likely

When to Refer

Immediate Transfer:

1. Tibial plateau fracture with significant displacement or neurovascular compromise
2. Open fracture or knee dislocation
3. Irreducible patellar dislocation
4. Suspected multi-ligament injury with unstable joint

Urgent Referral (1–3 days):

1. Reduced patellar dislocation
2. Confirmed tibial plateau fracture (non-displaced)
3. Persistent knee instability or large effusion

Routine Follow-up:

1. Mild sprains or suspected meniscal injuries
2. Follow-up in 7–10 days for reassessment and physio referral

Admission Orders

1. Admit to Rural Medicine – Knee Injury Observation
2. Diagnosis: Tibial plateau fracture / Patellar dislocation (reduced)
3. Condition: Stable
4. Allergies: [Document here]

Orders:

1. Vitals q4h
2. Analgesia:
3. Acetaminophen 1000 mg PO q6h
4. Ibuprofen 400 mg PO q6h
5. Morphine 2–5 mg SC q4h PRN
6. Immobilization: Knee immobilizer or long leg splint
7. Imaging: X-ray or CT if available
8. Neurovascular checks q4h
9. Activity: Strict non-weight-bearing, crutches
10. Referral: Orthopedic surgery or outpatient sports medicine
11. Discharge Plan: Pain controlled, splint education, follow-up confirmed

Rural ER Pearls

1. Patellar dislocation is common in young athletes and often reducible in the ED.
2. Tibial plateau fractures may be subtle on X-ray—look for joint depression or effusion.
3. Do not miss peroneal nerve palsy in knee trauma—check foot dorsiflexion.
4. Ligament testing is unreliable in the acute phase due to guarding and pain.
5. Use Ottawa Knee Rules to guide imaging decisions in blunt trauma.

CHAPTER 42
Patellar Dislocation and Patellar Fractures

Introduction

Patellar injuries, including dislocations and fractures, are relatively common in rural emergency departments, often resulting from direct trauma or twisting injuries. Lateral patellar dislocation is most common and may be associated with ligamentous injury. Patellar fractures can be transverse, vertical, comminuted, or osteochondral, and they require prompt recognition to preserve knee function. Early immobilization, reduction of dislocations, and appropriate referral are critical to preventing chronic instability or loss of knee extension.

Assessment

History:

1. Mechanism: direct blow, twisting injury, sudden quadriceps contraction
2. Inability to extend knee or bear weight
3. History of previous patellar instability
4. Audible pop at time of injury

Physical Exam:

1. Visible lateral displacement (in dislocation)
2. Swelling and hemarthrosis
3. Tenderness over patella and retinaculum
4. Palpable defect if fracture is displaced
5. Assess extensor mechanism: patient unable to straight leg raise if tendon disrupted
6. Neurovascular exam: popliteal pulse, distal sensation

Imaging:

1. X-ray knee (AP, lateral, and sunrise views)
2. Dislocation: patella displaced laterally on sunrise view
3. Fracture: assess fracture pattern, displacement, and comminution
4. Consider MRI if recurrent dislocations or suspected osteochondral injury

Management

Patellar Dislocation:

1. Provide analgesia and gentle reduction: extend knee while applying medial pressure to patella
2. Immobilize in extension with knee immobilizer or posterior splint
3. Encourage early range-of-motion after initial immobilization period
4. Arrange physiotherapy for quadriceps strengthening

Patellar Fractures:

1. Non-displaced: immobilization in extension, weight bearing as tolerated
2. Displaced (>2–3 mm separation or articular step-off): urgent orthopedic referral for surgical fixation

General Principles:

1. Ice, compression, elevation to reduce swelling
2. Analgesia: acetaminophen, NSAIDs, opioids for severe pain
3. Do not delay reduction if neurovascular compromise present

When to Refer

Immediate Transfer:

1. Open fracture
2. Irreducible dislocation
3. Neurovascular compromise

Urgent Referral (1–3 days):

1. Displaced fractures
2. Associated osteochondral fragments
3. Recurrent dislocations requiring surgical stabilization

Routine Follow-up:

1. First-time dislocation, successfully reduced, with no large fracture fragment
2. Non-displaced fracture managed conservatively

Admission Orders

1. Admit to Rural Medicine – Patellar Injury Observation
2. Diagnosis: Lateral patellar dislocation / Non-displaced patellar fracture
3. Condition: Stable
4. Allergies: [Document here]

Orders:

1. Vitals q4h
2. Analgesia:
3. Acetaminophen 1000 mg PO q6h
4. Ibuprofen 400 mg PO q6h
5. Morphine 2–5 mg SC q4h PRN
6. Immobilization: Knee immobilizer in full extension
7. Ice and elevate limb
8. Imaging: Repeat X-ray post-reduction if applicable

9. Neurovascular checks q4h
10. Referral: Orthopedic surgery as indicated
11. Discharge Plan: Pain controlled, immobilizer education, follow-up arranged

Rural ER Pearls

1. Always assess for osteochondral fragments after patellar dislocation
2. Early physiotherapy reduces recurrence risk in first-time dislocations
3. Do not miss quadriceps or patellar tendon rupture in the setting of patellar fracture
4. Lateral dislocation is most common; medial dislocation is rare and usually post-surgical

CHAPTER 43
Patellar Tendon Rupture

Introduction

Patellar tendon rupture is a serious knee injury that typically occurs in individuals under 40 years old, often during sports or activities involving forceful jumping or sudden changes in direction. It results in disruption of the knee's extensor mechanism, preventing active extension. Prompt diagnosis and referral for surgical repair are critical to restore function and prevent long-term disability.

Assessment

History:

1. Mechanism: sudden, forceful contraction of quadriceps with knee flexed (e.g., jumping, landing, stumbling)
2. Sudden anterior knee pain
3. Inability to straighten the knee or walk normally
4. Possible history of tendonitis, steroid injections, or systemic disease

Physical Exam:

1. Swelling and tenderness just below the patella
2. Palpable gap between patella and tibial tubercle
3. Patella alta (high-riding patella) on inspection
4. Inability to perform straight leg raise
5. Assess for associated injuries and perform neurovascular exam

Imaging:

1. X-ray knee (AP and lateral views): may show patella alta
2. Ultrasound: confirms tendon discontinuity

   3. MRI: gold standard if available, useful in partial tears

Management

General Approach:

   1. Immobilize knee in full extension with knee immobilizer or posterior splint
   2. Analgesia: acetaminophen, NSAIDs, opioids for severe pain
   3. Ice and elevate limb to reduce swelling

Complete Rupture:

   1. Requires urgent orthopedic referral for surgical repair
   2. Keep patient non-weight-bearing until surgical assessment

Partial Rupture:

   1. May be managed with immobilization and physiotherapy if extensor mechanism remains intact
   2. Early orthopedic review recommended

When to Refer

Immediate Transfer:

   1. Complete rupture with loss of active extension
   2. Open tendon injury
   3. Associated fractures

Urgent Referral (within 1–3 days):

   1. Partial rupture with significant functional limitation
   2. Delayed presentations with persistent weakness

Admission Orders

1. Admit to Rural Medicine – Patellar Tendon Rupture
2. Diagnosis: Complete patellar tendon rupture
3. Condition: Stable
4. Allergies: [Document here]

Orders:

1. Vitals q4h
2. Analgesia:
3. Acetaminophen 1000 mg PO q6h
4. Ibuprofen 400 mg PO q6h
5. Morphine 2–5 mg SC q4h PRN
6. Immobilization: Knee immobilizer in full extension
7. Ice and elevate limb
8. Imaging: Knee X-ray, ultrasound if available
9. Neurovascular checks q4h
10. Referral: Orthopedic surgery as indicated
11. Discharge Plan: Pain controlled, splint education, follow-up arranged

Rural ER Pearls

1. Patella alta on X-ray is suggestive of patellar tendon rupture
2. Differentiate from quadriceps tendon rupture (which shows patella baja)
3. Always check for associated ligamentous injuries in sports trauma
4. Early surgical repair offers the best outcomes

CHAPTER 44
Quadriceps Tendon Rupture

Introduction

Quadriceps tendon rupture is an uncommon but serious injury, typically seen in middle-aged or older adults, often with predisposing factors such as chronic kidney disease, diabetes, or corticosteroid use. It usually occurs during forceful contraction of the quadriceps muscle against resistance, such as when trying to prevent a fall. Prompt recognition and surgical referral are essential to restore knee extension and function.

Assessment

History:

1. Mechanism: sudden forceful quadriceps contraction, fall, stumble, or jump landing
2. Sudden onset anterior knee pain
3. Inability to extend the knee actively
4. History of systemic disease or corticosteroid use

Physical Exam:

1. Swelling and tenderness superior to patella
2. Palpable gap above patella in complete rupture
3. Inability to perform straight leg raise
4. Bruising and hematoma formation
5. Assess for associated patellar fracture
6. Neurovascular exam: distal pulses and sensation

Imaging:

1. X-ray knee: may show low-lying patella (patella baja) in complete rupture
2. Ultrasound: useful in rural settings to confirm tendon discontinuity
3. MRI: gold standard for diagnosis if available

Management

General Approach:

1. Immobilize knee in full extension with knee immobilizer or posterior slab
2. Analgesia: acetaminophen, NSAIDs, opioids if severe pain
3. Ice and elevate limb to reduce swelling

Complete Rupture:

1. Requires urgent orthopedic referral for surgical repair
2. Keep patient non-weight-bearing until assessed by orthopedics

Partial Rupture:

1. May be managed with immobilization and physiotherapy in select cases
2. Early orthopedic review still recommended

When to Refer

Immediate Transfer:

1. Complete rupture with loss of active knee extension
2. Open tendon injury
3. Associated patellar fracture

Urgent Referral (within 1–3 days):

1. Partial rupture with significant functional limitation
2. Delayed presentations with persistent extension weakness

Admission Orders

1. Admit to Rural Medicine – Quadriceps Tendon Rupture
2. Diagnosis: Complete quadriceps tendon rupture
3. Condition: Stable
4. Allergies: [Document here]

Orders:

1. Vitals q4h
2. Analgesia:
3. Acetaminophen 1000 mg PO q6h
4. Ibuprofen 400 mg PO q6h
5. Morphine 2–5 mg SC q4h PRN
6. Immobilization: Knee immobilizer in full extension
7. Ice and elevate limb
8. Imaging: Knee X-ray, ultrasound if available
9. Neurovascular checks q4h
10. Referral: Orthopedic surgery as indicated
11. Discharge Plan: Pain controlled, splint education, follow-up arranged

Rural ER Pearls

1. Always compare with the opposite knee when assessing for tendon defects
2. Patella baja on X-ray suggests quadriceps tendon rupture
3. High index of suspicion in older adults with sudden knee pain and inability to extend
4. Early surgical repair offers best functional outcomes

LEG: TIBIA & FIBULA

CHAPTER 45
Tibial and Fibular Shaft Fractures

Introduction

Tibial and fibular shaft fractures are common lower limb injuries that occur from both high-energy trauma (e.g., motor vehicle collisions) and low-energy mechanisms (e.g., falls in osteoporotic patients). The tibia is particularly vulnerable as it has minimal soft tissue coverage, making open fractures and compartment syndrome significant concerns in rural emergency settings.

Assessment

History:

1. Mechanism: direct blow, twisting, fall, MVC
2. Pain severity, inability to bear weight
3. Paresthesia, numbness, or muscle weakness
4. Time since injury
5. Medications: anticoagulants, osteoporosis treatment

Physical Exam:

1. Visible deformity, bruising, or swelling
2. Open wounds (check for open fracture)
3. Tenderness along tibial shaft
4. Assess compartments for tightness or pain with passive stretch (compartment syndrome)

Neurovascular exam:

1. Dorsalis pedis, posterior tibial pulses
2. Sensory: superficial peroneal and tibial nerves
3. Motor: dorsiflexion, plantarflexion

Imaging:

1. X-ray of tibia/fibula (AP and lateral), include ankle and knee
2. CT if joint involvement or subtle fracture suspected

Management

Initial Management:

1. Immobilize with long leg posterior slab or padded board splint
2. Elevate and apply ice
3. IV analgesia: opioids, acetaminophen, NSAIDs
4. Tetanus update and IV antibiotics if open fracture
5. Assess for compartment syndrome

Open Fractures:

1. Do not close wounds
2. Cover with moist sterile dressing
3. Administer broad-spectrum IV antibiotics (cefazolin +/- gentamicin/metronidazole)

Compartment Syndrome:

1. Monitor closely, especially in high-energy injuries or tight casts/splints
2. Pain out of proportion, pain on passive stretch, firm compartments
3. Emergent referral if suspected

Surgical Referral:

1. Most tibial shaft fractures require ORIF or intramedullary nailing

When to Refer

Immediate Transfer:

1. Open fracture
2. Suspected compartment syndrome
3. Neurovascular compromise
4. Segmental or comminuted fracture
5. Polytrauma

Urgent Referral (within 24–48 hours):

1. Closed, displaced fracture in stable patient
2. Isolated tibia fracture with good neurovascular status

Routine Follow-up:

1. Non-displaced, isolated fibular fracture
2. Follow-up in 7–10 days for reassessment and repeat imaging

Admission Orders

1. Admit to Rural Medicine – Tibial/Fibular Shaft Fracture
2. Diagnosis: Displaced tibial shaft fracture
3. Condition: Stable
4. Allergies: [Document here]

Orders:

1. Vitals q2h for first 12h, then q4h
2. IV fluids: NS at 100 mL/hr
3. Analgesia:
4. Acetaminophen 1000 mg PO q6h
5. Morphine 2–5 mg IV q4h PRN
6. Immobilization: Long leg posterior slab, elevate limb
7. Antibiotics: Cefazolin 2 g IV q8h (add gentamicin/metronidazole if open)

8. Tetanus prophylaxis PRN
9. Neurovascular checks and compartment checks q2h x 12h, then q4h
10. Imaging: X-rays of tibia/fibula including joints
11. Referral: Orthopedic consultation and transfer if needed
12. Discharge Plan: Pain controlled, neurovascularly intact, follow-up/transfer arranged

Rural ER Pearls

1. Always include the knee and ankle in imaging of tibia/fibula shaft injuries.
2. Open tibial fractures require early antibiotics and sterile dressing—not closure.
3. Compartment syndrome can develop even in closed fractures — monitor closely.
4. Fibular shaft fractures alone are often stable but can signal ankle instability — assess proximally and distally.
5. Elevate and immobilize early to minimize pain and swelling.

ANKLE, FOOT & TOES (INCL. ACHILLES)

CHAPTER 46
Ankle Fractures

Introduction

Ankle fractures are among the most frequently encountered orthopedic injuries in rural emergency departments. These injuries vary from simple lateral malleolus fractures to complex bimalleolar or trimalleolar fractures. The Weber classification system helps guide management based on the level of the fibular fracture in relation to the syndesmosis. Early immobilization, accurate classification, and appropriate referral are essential for preventing long-term complications like instability or arthritis.

Assessment

History:

1. Mechanism: twisting injury, fall, sports trauma
2. Inability to bear weight or walk
3. Previous ankle injuries or surgeries
4. Pain location: lateral, medial, posterior

Physical Exam:

1. Swelling, bruising, deformity of ankle
2. Tenderness at malleoli, base of 5th metatarsal, navicular
3. Assess for open wounds or tenting skin
4. Neurovascular exam:
5. Dorsalis pedis and posterior tibial pulses
6. Sensory and motor function in foot

Imaging:

1. X-ray ankle (AP, lateral, mortise views)
2. Ottawa Ankle Rules:

3. Bone tenderness at malleoli
4. Inability to bear weight immediately and in ED

Weber Classification:

1. Weber A: below syndesmosis
2. Weber B: at syndesmosis
3. Weber C: above syndesmosis (unstable, often needs surgery)
4. Evaluate medial clear space and mortise widening

Management

General Approach:

1. RICE: rest, ice, compression, elevation
2. Immobilization with posterior slab or stirrup splint
3. Analgesia: NSAIDs, acetaminophen, opioids if needed
4. Elevate limb to reduce swelling

Closed Fractures:

1. Weber A: often stable, treated with splint and outpatient follow-up
2. Weber B: variable stability, may require surgical referral
3. Weber C: unstable, surgical fixation indicated

Reduction:

1. Attempt gentle closed reduction for dislocated or misaligned ankle
2. Post-reduction X-ray to confirm alignment

Open Fractures:

1. IV antibiotics, sterile dressing, urgent referral

Do Not:

1. Ignore medial pain or deltoid ligament tenderness—it may indicate bimalleolar injury
2. Delay reduction if there is neurovascular compromise

When to Refer

Immediate Transfer:

1. Open fracture
2. Neurovascular compromise
3. Dislocation not reducible in ED
4. Trimalleolar fracture or unstable bimalleolar fracture

Urgent Referral (1–3 days):

1. Weber C fracture (above syndesmosis)
2. Weber B fracture with mortise widening or deltoid ligament involvement

Routine Follow-up:

1. Isolated Weber A fracture with normal mortise
2. Non-displaced Weber B fracture with intact medial structures
3. Follow-up in 7–10 days for reassessment

Admission Orders

1. Admit to Rural Medicine – Ankle Fracture Observation
2. Diagnosis: Weber B lateral malleolus fracture
3. Condition: Stable
4. Allergies: [Document here]

Orders:

1. Vitals q4h
2. Analgesia:
3. Acetaminophen 1000 mg PO q6h
4. Ibuprofen 400 mg PO q6h
5. Morphine 2–5 mg SC q4h PRN
6. Immobilization: Posterior slab or stirrup splint
7. Elevate limb, ice pack application
8. Imaging: Repeat X-ray post-reduction if applicable
9. Neurovascular checks q4h
10. Tetanus and antibiotics if open fracture
11. Referral: Orthopedic surgery referral as indicated
12. Discharge Plan: Pain controlled, splint education, follow-up arranged

Rural ER Pearls

1. Use the Weber classification to guide urgency of referral.
2. Not all Weber B fractures are surgical—but beware of mortise widening.
3. Always examine and image the entire ankle mortise and syndesmosis.
4. Beware of Maisonneuve fracture: proximal fibula fracture with ankle instability.
5. Prompt reduction reduces risk of skin necrosis in dislocated ankles.

CHAPTER 47
Foot Fractures

Introduction

Foot fractures are common injuries seen in rural emergency settings, frequently caused by falls, crush injuries, or twisting mechanisms. They include metatarsal fractures, calcaneal fractures, and Lisfranc injuries. Some fractures are easily missed on initial presentation. Timely diagnosis, appropriate imaging, and immobilization are key to preventing long-term disability or chronic pain.

Assessment

History:

1. Mechanism: direct blow, fall from height, crush injury, twist
2. Weight-bearing ability post-injury
3. Footwear at time of injury
4. Location of pain and swelling

Physical Exam:

1. Inspect for swelling, bruising, deformity
2. Palpate for tenderness over:
3. Metatarsals (especially base of 5th)
4. Midfoot (Lisfranc joint)
5. Heel (calcaneus)
6. Assess for plantar ecchymosis (suggests Lisfranc injury)
7. Squeeze test for midfoot instability
8. Neurovascular exam: cap refill, dorsal and plantar sensation

Imaging:

1. X-ray foot (AP, lateral, oblique views)
2. Weight-bearing films if Lisfranc injury suspected
3. CT if subtle fracture or comminution suspected (especially calcaneus)

Management

Metatarsal Fractures:

1. Non-displaced: hard-soled shoe or posterior splint, weight-bearing as tolerated
2. 5th metatarsal base (Jones fracture): often non-weight-bearing, surgical consult
3. Displaced fractures: splint and refer for surgical opinion

Calcaneal Fractures:

1. High suspicion with fall from height and heel pain
2. Immobilize and keep non-weight-bearing
3. CT to assess for intra-articular involvement
4. Watch for compartment syndrome in foot

Lisfranc Injuries:

1. Often subtle on X-ray
2. Plantar ecchymosis is a key finding
3. If suspected, immobilize and keep non-weight-bearing
4. Surgical referral mandatory

General:

1. Posterior slab splint or walking boot
2. Elevate and ice
3. NSAIDs or opioids as needed
4. Tetanus and antibiotics if open fracture

When to Refer

Immediate Transfer:

1. Open fracture
2. Neurovascular compromise
3. Compartment syndrome
4. Comminuted calcaneal fracture with skin tenting
5. Displaced Lisfranc injury

Urgent Referral (1–3 days):

1. Jones fracture of 5th metatarsal
2. Displaced or multiple metatarsal fractures
3. Suspected Lisfranc injury with stable vitals

Routine Follow-up:

1. Non-displaced metatarsal shaft fracture
2. Calcaneal avulsion fractures
3. Follow-up in 7–10 days with repeat imaging if needed

Admission Orders

1. Admit to Rural Medicine – Foot Fracture Observation
2. Diagnosis: Displaced 5th metatarsal fracture / Suspected Lisfranc injury
3. Condition: Stable
4. Allergies: [Document here]

Orders:

1. Vitals q4h
2. Analgesia:
3. Acetaminophen 1000 mg PO q6h
4. Ibuprofen 400 mg PO q6h
5. Morphine 2–5 mg SC q4h PRN
6. Immobilization: Posterior slab or walking boot

7. Activity: Strict non-weight-bearing with crutches
8. Imaging: Foot X-ray (weight-bearing if Lisfranc suspected), CT if available
9. Neurovascular checks q4h
10. Elevate foot above heart level
11. Referral: Orthopedic or podiatry if available
12. Discharge Plan: Stable, follow-up confirmed, splint education provided

Rural ER Pearls

1. Plantar ecchymosis is pathognomonic for Lisfranc injury.
2. Never miss a Jones fracture — delayed healing is common.
3. Calcaneal fractures are associated with lumbar spine injuries — check back pain.
4. Weight-bearing films increase sensitivity for detecting Lisfranc disruption.
5. Elevation and proper splinting help reduce swelling and pain early on.

CHAPTER 48
Toe Injuries

Introduction

Toe injuries are common presentations in rural emergency departments, often resulting from direct trauma, stubbing, or crush mechanisms. While many toe injuries are minor, appropriate assessment is necessary to rule out open fractures, joint dislocations, and subungual hematomas that require drainage or nailbed repair.

Assessment

History:

1. Mechanism: stubbed toe, crush injury, dropped object
2. Pain, swelling, bleeding
3. History of diabetes, peripheral neuropathy, or anticoagulant use

Physical Exam:

1. Inspection: deformity, swelling, open wounds, nailbed damage
2. Palpation: tenderness, step-offs
3. Assess joint alignment and range of motion
4. Neurovascular exam: capillary refill, distal sensation

Imaging:

1. Toe/finger X-ray (AP, lateral, oblique)
2. Assess for fracture displacement, intra-articular involvement, or dislocation

Management

Toe Fractures:

1. Non-displaced: buddy taping to adjacent toe, hard-soled shoe
2. Displaced: digital block and closed reduction if trained
3. Intra-articular or unstable fractures: splint and refer
4. Open fracture: irrigate, dress, antibiotics, tetanus, refer

Toe Dislocations:

1. Often at PIP or DIP joints
2. Perform closed reduction after digital block
3. Post-reduction X-ray to confirm alignment
4. Immobilize with buddy taping

Subungual Hematoma:

1. If <25% and painless: observe
2. If >25% or painful: trephination with cautery or sterile needle
3. Remove nail if underlying laceration suspected (especially if nail edge disrupted)

Wound Care:

1. Clean with saline
2. Apply antibiotic ointment and sterile dressing
3. Update tetanus status

When to Refer

Immediate Transfer:

1. Open fracture with significant soft tissue loss
2. Nailbed laceration with exposed matrix
3. Dislocation not reducible

4. Compromised perfusion or sensation

Urgent Referral (1–3 days):

1. Displaced or intra-articular toe fracture
2. Suspected osteomyelitis (especially in diabetics)
3. Large subungual hematoma with nailbed laceration

Routine Follow-up:

1. Non-displaced toe fractures with intact neurovascular exam
2. Subungual hematoma <25% with minimal symptoms
3. Follow-up in 7–10 days to monitor healing

Admission Orders

1. Admit to Rural Medicine – Toe Injury Observation
2. Diagnosis: Displaced second toe fracture / Subungual hematoma
3. Condition: Stable
4. Allergies: [Document here]

Orders:

1. Vitals q4h
2. Analgesia:
3. Acetaminophen 1000 mg PO q6h
4. Ibuprofen 400 mg PO q6h
5. Immobilization: Buddy taping or toe splint
6. Imaging: Toe X-ray (repeat if post-reduction)
7. Wound care: Irrigate and dress open wounds
8. Antibiotics: Cephalexin 500 mg PO q6h if open fracture
9. Tetanus update if required
10. Activity: Crutches if unable to bear weight
11. Referral: Podiatry or orthopedic consultation as indicated

12. Discharge Plan: Pain controlled, instructions provided, follow-up confirmed

Rural ER Pearls

1. Most toe fractures are managed conservatively with buddy taping.
2. Always rule out open fracture in crush injuries.
3. Trephination is effective and safe for painful subungual hematomas.
4. Remove the nail only if the nailbed is visibly disrupted or floating.
5. Diabetic patients with toe trauma require close monitoring for infection or ischemia.
6. .

CHAPTER 49
Achilles Tendon Rupture

Introduction

Achilles tendon rupture is a common injury in middle-aged patients engaging in sudden athletic activity, such as jumping or sprinting. Early recognition and immobilization are key to optimizing functional recovery. In rural emergency settings, clinical diagnosis is often sufficient and early referral to orthopedics is recommended for surgical versus conservative management.

Assessment

History:

1. Sudden "pop" or "kick" sensation in the heel
2. Immediate difficulty walking or pushing off foot
3. Common in recreational athletes over age 30
4. May have history of tendonitis, fluoroquinolone or steroid use

Physical Exam:

1. Swelling and bruising in posterior ankle
2. Palpable gap in tendon
3. Positive **Thompson test**: no plantarflexion when calf squeezed
4. Weak or absent active plantarflexion
5. Compare to uninjured side
6. Check neurovascular status (cap refill, sensation, pulses)

Imaging:

1. Clinical diagnosis is often sufficient
2. Ultrasound (if available) can confirm rupture

3. MRI usually reserved for uncertain cases or pre-op planning

Management

Initial ED Management:

1. Immobilize ankle in plantarflexion (equinus position) using posterior slab
2. Non-weight-bearing with crutches
3. Elevate leg and apply ice
4. Analgesia: acetaminophen, NSAIDs, opioids PRN
5. Do not dorsiflex foot or allow weight-bearing

Definitive Management:

1. All patients require orthopedic referral
2. Operative vs non-operative management depends on age, activity level, and rupture extent
3. Early functional rehab improves outcomes in both approaches

Do Not:

1. Allow ambulation without protection
2. Stretch or dorsiflex the foot acutely
3. Delay immobilization

When to Refer

Immediate Transfer:

1. Open Achilles rupture (rare)
2. Combined injury with fracture or neurovascular compromise

Urgent Referral (within 1–3 days):

1. All suspected Achilles tendon ruptures
2. Large partial tears in athletes or active adults

Routine Follow-up:

1. Minor partial tears in low-demand patients (rare)
2. Follow-up in 5–7 days with orthopedics or sports medicine

Admission Orders

1. Admit to Rural Medicine – Achilles Tendon Rupture
2. Diagnosis: Suspected complete Achilles tendon rupture
3. Condition: Stable
4. Allergies: [Document here]

Orders:

1. Vitals q4h
2. Analgesia:
3. Acetaminophen 1000 mg PO q6h
4. Ibuprofen 400 mg PO q6h
5. Morphine 2–5 mg SC q4h PRN
6. Immobilization: Posterior slab in plantarflexion
7. Activity: Strict non-weight-bearing with crutches
8. Imaging: Ultrasound if available
9. Referral: Orthopedic consultation
10. Discharge Plan: Stable, pain controlled, splint education provided, follow-up confirmed

Rural ER Pearls

1. The Thompson test is highly sensitive and specific—use it routinely.
2. Fluoroquinolones and corticosteroids increase rupture risk.
3. Immobilization in plantarflexion is critical to tendon healing.
4. Missed ruptures can present later with persistent weakness and gait abnormalities.
5. Early rehab protocols are evolving—consult orthopedic guidelines in your region.

TENDONS & SOFT-TISSUE (GENERAL)

CHAPTER 50
Tendon Injuries

Introduction

Tendon injuries of the hand are serious injuries that can significantly impair hand function if not promptly identified and treated. Flexor tendon injuries are typically more severe and require urgent surgical repair, while extensor tendon injuries may be managed conservatively depending on location and severity. In rural emergency settings, accurate identification of the tendon zone involved and timely referral are crucial.

Assessment

History:

1. Mechanism: laceration, crush injury, sharp objects, glass, power tools
2. Hand dominance
3. Finger involved and position at injury
4. Tetanus immunization status

Physical Exam:

1. Assess for open wounds, depth, and visible tendon
2. Test active flexion and extension of all joints (DIP, PIP, MCP)
3. Check for dropped finger, loss of flexion, or extension lag

Neurovascular status:

1. Capillary refill
2. Sensation (2-point discrimination)
3. Median, ulnar, and radial nerve testing

Imaging:

1. X-rays if bony involvement or foreign body is suspected
2. Ultrasound (if available) to visualize tendon discontinuity in closed injuries

Management

General Principles:

1. Irrigation and clean dressing
2. Tetanus prophylaxis and antibiotics for open wounds
3. Immobilization in position of function using volar splint
4. Avoid probing wounds which may worsen damage

Flexor Tendon Injuries:

1. Always refer to hand surgery
2. Zone II injuries (no man's land) have high complication risk
3. Immobilize and elevate

Extensor Tendon Injuries:

1. Zone I (mallet finger): stack splint for 6–8 weeks
2. Zone III (boutonnière): extension splint PIP joint
3. Zone VI–VIII: lacerations over dorsum require splint and referral

Surgical Referral Indications:

1. All flexor tendon lacerations
2. Complex or multi-tendon injuries
3. Injuries with neurovascular compromise
4. Open wounds with exposed tendon or bone

When to Refer

Immediate Transfer:

1. Complete flexor tendon laceration
2. Combined neurovascular injury
3. Contaminated or infected deep wound
4. Multiple finger involvement or crush injury

Urgent Referral (1–3 days):

1. Extensor tendon laceration with partial rupture
2. Mallet finger not amenable to splinting
3. Suspected tendon rupture with closed injury and functional deficit

Routine Follow-up:

1. Minor extensor injuries in stable alignment
2. Well-controlled mallet finger with good compliance
3. Arrange splint checks and follow-up in 5–7 days

Admission Orders

1. Admit to Rural Medicine – Tendon Injury Observation
2. Diagnosis: Flexor tendon laceration / Extensor tendon injury
3. Condition: Stable
4. Allergies: [Document here]

Orders:

1. Vitals q4h
2. Analgesia:
3. Acetaminophen 1000 mg PO q6h PRN
4. Ibuprofen 400 mg PO q6h PRN
5. Morphine 2–5 mg SC q4h PRN for severe pain
6. Immobilization: Volar splint in position of function

7. Wound care: Clean dressing, irrigation as needed
8. Tetanus update if required
9. Antibiotics: Cefazolin 1 g IV q8h or PO cephalexin if outpatient
10. Neurovascular checks q4h
11. Activity: Hand elevation, non-weight-bearing
12. Referral: Fax to plastic/hand surgeon
13. Discharge Plan: Stable, wound clean, follow-up arranged

Rural ER Pearls

1. Always test all finger joints for flexion and extension in hand injuries.
2. Zone II flexor injuries ("no man's land") have the worst prognosis and need expert repair.
3. Mallet finger requires strict 24/7 splinting—removal for even a second can disrupt healing.
4. Suspect closed tendon rupture in patients with inability to flex/extend despite minimal trauma.
5. Don't forget antibiotics and tetanus in all open tendon lacerations.

CHAPTER 51
Midshaft Humerus Fractures

Introduction

Midshaft humerus fractures account for approximately 3% of all fractures and are often caused by falls, direct trauma, or motor vehicle accidents. They may be associated with radial nerve injury and require careful neurovascular assessment. In rural settings, most can be managed conservatively with proper immobilization and follow-up.

Assessment

History:

1. Mechanism: fall on outstretched hand, direct blow, twisting injury
2. Dominant arm involved?
3. Associated numbness or wrist drop?
4. Medical history: osteoporosis, anticoagulants, malignancy

Physical Exam:

1. Visible deformity or angulation at the mid-arm
2. Swelling, tenderness, crepitus over the humerus
3. Assess radial nerve: wrist/finger extension, dorsal hand sensation
4. Assess median, ulnar nerve and distal pulses
5. Skin inspection for open fracture signs

Imaging:

1. X-ray humerus (AP and lateral views of entire humerus including shoulder and elbow)
2. Consider additional shoulder/elbow views if pain present

Management

Conservative (most closed, non-comminuted fractures):

1. Immobilization with a coaptation splint or functional brace
2. Analgesia: acetaminophen, NSAIDs, opioids short-term if severe
3. Elevation and ice for swelling
4. Begin pendulum exercises after 7–10 days

Surgical Referral Indications:

1. Open fracture
2. Vascular injury
3. Segmental or comminuted fracture
4. Pathologic fracture (e.g., malignancy)
5. Failure to maintain alignment or unacceptable angulation
6. Radial nerve palsy with fracture (controversial; monitor vs explore)

When to Refer

Immediate Transfer:

1. Open fracture
2. Suspected vascular injury
3. Progressive or complete radial nerve palsy with wrist drop

Urgent Orthopedic Referral (1–3 days):

1. Severely displaced or angulated fractures
2. Comminuted or segmental fracture
3. Suspected pathologic fracture (e.g., history of cancer)

Routine Follow-up:

1. Stable, closed, non-displaced fracture
2. Radial nerve palsy with spontaneous function
3. Follow-up in 7–10 days with X-ray and orthopedic consult

Admission Orders

1. Admit to Rural Medicine – Midshaft Humerus Fracture
2. Diagnosis: Closed midshaft humerus fracture
3. Condition: Stable
4. Allergies: [Document here]

Orders:

1. Vitals q4h
2. Analgesia:
3. Acetaminophen 1000 mg PO q6h PRN
4. Ibuprofen 400 mg PO q6h PRN
5. Morphine 2–5 mg SC q4h PRN for severe pain
6. Immobilization: Apply coaptation splint and sling
7. Imaging: Repeat X-ray if worsening pain or neurovascular signs
8. Neurovascular checks q4h (focus on radial nerve)
9. Activity: Bedrest with sling support
10. Referral: Fax referral to orthopedic surgery
11. Discharge Plan: Stable vitals, pain control, clear discharge instructions, sling care

Rural ER Pearls

1. Always check and document radial nerve function—wrist drop may be first clue.
2. Most midshaft humerus fractures can be treated non-operatively.
3. Coaptation splint is preferred in acute phase to reduce swelling before switching to functional brace.
4. Monitor for signs of compartment syndrome in high-energy trauma.
5. Radial nerve palsy present at initial assessment may resolve spontaneously in weeks—observation often appropriate.

REFERENCES

This list includes publicly available, non-subscription medical guidelines and clinical reference sources. These resources were cited for general guidance only. No copyrighted material, charts, or proprietary algorithms have been reproduced. All references are legally accessible for citation.

Orthopedics (Open Access)

- British Orthopaedic Association (BOA) — BOAST Standards for Trauma Care. https://www.boa.ac.uk — Accessed August 2025.
- NICE — Fractures (non-complex); Fractures (complex); Hip fracture management (current versions). https://www.nice.org.uk — Accessed August 2025.
- Orthopaedic Trauma Association (OTA) — Educational resources & fracture classification overview. https://ota.org — Accessed August 2025.
- Canadian Orthopaedic Association (COA) — Position statements and practice resources. https://coa-aco.org — Accessed August 2025.
- Canadian Association of Emergency Physicians (CAEP) — Procedural Sedation Guidelines. https://caep.ca — Accessed August 2025.
- American College of Emergency Physicians (ACEP) — Procedural Sedation in the ED (clinical policy/guidance). https://www.acep.org — Accessed August 2025.
- Thrombosis Canada — VTE prophylaxis in orthopedic surgery & perioperative anticoagulation guidance. https://thrombosiscanada.ca — Accessed August 2025.
- Infectious Diseases Society of America (IDSA) — Skin & Soft Tissue Infections Guideline (2023 update); plus

Osteomyelitis/Prosthetic Joint Infection guidelines. https://www.idsociety.org — Accessed August 2025.

- Public Health Agency of Canada — Canadian Immunization Guide (tetanus in wound management). https://www.canada.ca — Accessed August 2025.
- Centers for Disease Control and Prevention (CDC) — Tetanus prophylaxis in wound management. https://www.cdc.gov — Accessed August 2025.
- American College of Radiology (ACR) — Appropriateness Criteria® for Musculoskeletal Imaging & Acute Trauma. https://www.acr.org — Accessed August 2025.
- Ottawa Hospital Research Institute (OHRI) — Clinical Decision Rules (Ottawa Ankle, Ottawa Knee; Canadian C-Spine Rule). https://www.ohri.ca — Accessed August 2025.
- Osteoporosis Canada — Clinical Practice Guidelines. https://osteoporosis.ca — Accessed August 2025.
- Canadian Task Force on Preventive Health Care (CTFPHC) — Screening & preventive care recommendations relevant to MSK health. https://canadiantaskforce.ca — Accessed August 2025.

Further Reading (open web — do not reproduce figures/tables)

- OrthoBullets — Orthopedic condition and trauma summaries. https://www.orthobullets.com — Accessed August 2025.

www.ingramcontent.com/pod-product-compliance
Lightning Source LLC
Chambersburg PA
CBHW040920210326

41597CB00030B/5135